Health
Policymaking
in the
United States

Health Policymaking in the United States

Beaufort B. Longest, Jr.

AUPHA Press/Health Administration Press
Ann Arbor, Michigan   1994

98 97 96   5 4 3

Library of Congress Cataloging-in-Publication Data

Longest, Beaufort B.
  Health policymaking in the United States / Beaufort B. Longest, Jr.
    p.   cm.
  Includes bibliographical references and index.
  ISBN 1-56793-017-4
  1. Medical policy—United States—Decision making. 2. Health planning—United States. 3. Medical laws and legislation—United States. 4. Policy sciences—Methodology. I. Title.
  RA395.A3L66   1994   362.1'0973—dc20   94-18790 CIP

The paper used in this publication meets the minimum requirements of American National Standard for Information Sciences—Permanence of Paper for Printed Library Materials, ANSI Z39.48-1984.

Health Administration Press
A division of the Foundation
  of the American College of
  Healthcare Executives
1021 East Huron Street
Ann Arbor, Michigan 48104-1628
(313) 764-1380

Association of University Programs
  in Health Administration
1911 North Fort Myer Drive, Suite 503
Arlington, Virginia 22209
(703) 524-5500

For Carolyn

Though a myriad leagues of hill and stream
divide them, hearts truly in touch
do not find the way to each other long.

Zeami, *Takasago*

Contents

List of Abbreviations

AAFP	American Academy of Family Physicians
AAMC	Association of American Medical Colleges
AARP	American Association of Retired Persons
ACEHSA	Accrediting Commission on Education for Health Services Administration
ACGME	Accreditation Council for Graduate Medical Education
ACHE	American College of Healthcare Executives
ACP	American College of Physicians
ACS	American College of Surgeons
ADA	Americans With Disabilities Act
AFDC	Aid to Families With Dependent Children
AHA	American Hospital Association
AHCPR	Agency for Health Care Policy and Research
AMA	American Medical Association
ANA	American Nurses' Association
AUPHA	Association of University Programs in Health Administration
CBA	Cost-benefit analysis
CBO	Congressional Budget Office
CEA	Cost-effectiveness analysis
CERCLA	Comprehensive Environmental Response, Compensation, and Liability Act
COBRA	Consolidated Budget Reconciliation Act
CON	Certificate of need
COTH	Council of Teaching Hospitals
DEFRA	Deficit Reduction Act
DHEW	Department of Health, Education, and Welfare (now DHHS)
DHHS	Department of Health and Human Services

DO	Doctor of osteopathy
DOD	Department of Defense
DRG	Diagnosis-related groups
EEOC	Equal Employment Opportunity Commission
EMS	Emergency medical service
EPA	Environmental Protection Agency
EPL	Effective patient life
ERISA	Employee Retirement Income Security Act
ESRD	End-stage renal disease
FAHS	Federation of American Health Systems
FDA	Food and Drug Administration
FMG	Foreign medical graduate
GAO	General Accounting Office
GDP	Gross Domestic Product
GHAA	Group Health Association of America
HCFA	Health Care Financing Administration
HIAA	Health Insurance Association of America
HMO	Health maintenance organization
HSA	Health Systems Agency
ICF	Intermediate Care Facilities
JCAHO	Joint Commission on Accreditation of Healthcare Organizations
MAACs	Maximum allowable actual charges
MD	Medical doctor
MGMA	Medical Group Management Association
NASA	National Aeronautics and Space Administration
NCHSR	National Center for Health Services Research and Technology Assessment
NHSC	National Health Service Corps
NIH	National Institutes of Health
NLN	National League for Nursing
NPRM	Notice of Proposed Rulemaking
NRC	Nuclear Regulatory Commission
NSF	National Science Foundation
OBRA	Omnibus Budget Reconciliation Act
ODA	Orphan Drug Act
OMB	Office of Management and Budget
OSHA	Occupational Safety and Health Administration

PAC	Political action committee
PAR	Participating Physician and Supplier
PhRMA	Pharmaceutical Research and Manufacturers of America
PPRC	Physician Payment Review Commission
PPS	Prospective Payment System
PRO	Peer Review Organization
ProPac	Prospective Payment Assessment Commission
PSRO	Professional standards review organization
PTAC	Professional and technical advisory committees
RBRVS	Resource-based relative value scale
RN	Registered nurse
ROE	Return on equity
SHCC	State Health Coordinating Councils
SHPDA	State Health Planning and Development Agency
SNF	Skilled nursing facility
TEFRA	Tax Equity and Fiscal Responsibility Act
TSCA	Toxic Substances Control Act
VA	Veterans Affairs

Preface

Health policy occupies an unprecedented place on the domestic policy agenda in the United States as the twentieth century winds down. Driven by the intractable problem of escalating costs and continuing inequities in access to health care, the nation appears poised for major reform of its health policy, both at the federal level and in many of the states. Within the decade, we may see for the first time the formulation and implementation of a macro policy regarding health—a policy that seeks to both ensure universal access to health care services and to more rigorously control health expenditures. While the United States has lagged behind the other advanced democracies in developing a macro health policy, it has nevertheless evolved a vast array of policies pertaining to health. It formulates, implements, and modifies these policies within an intricately choreographed process. The purpose of this book is to provide those who have an interest in or a curiosity about health policy with a comprehensive model of this process.

The model of the health policymaking process, which forms the structure of this book, was developed for the benefit of my own health management and policy students. The fact that the model has proved useful as a framework for their consideration of the extraordinarily complicated process of health policymaking has stimulated me to present it to a broader audience through this book. The book will be useful for introductory courses in health policy as a means to provide students with an overview of the policymaking process. The model provides a framework that helps students put the various aspects of policymaking in perspective as they add to their knowledge of the process. Ultimately, it permits them to see the process as a set of highly interrelated phases of activity.

The model may also be useful to others who seek a better understanding of this process outside the classroom. Those involved in providing health care services or in producing resources used to create the services are directly affected by health policies. So too are those who utilize the services or pay for them. Importantly, a better understanding of the process through which health policies are made permits those affected by them to more effectively influence the policies and to more accurately predict their evolution and impacts. The model may even be useful to certain policymakers who, like all human beings, sometimes lose sight of the larger landscape of their work by becoming so intensely involved in its details.

In Chapter 1, "Health and Health Policy," health is broadly defined and shown to be determined by the physical, sociocultural, and economic environments in which people live; by their lifestyles and genetics; and by the health care system that serves them. Public policies are defined as authoritative decisions made in the legislative, executive, or judicial branches of government—decisions intended to direct or influence the actions, behaviors, or decisions of others. Health policies, in turn, are defined as public policies that pertain to or influence the pursuit of health. The breadth of the determinants of human health means that health policies span a wide range of issues, problems, and opportunities.

Chapter 2, "A Model of Public Policymaking for Health," contains a background explanation of the political market for health policies, including consideration of the demanders and suppliers of health policies in the United States. Power and influence within the political marketplace are explained and the key ethical issues that arise in this market are identified. An overview of the model of the policymaking process is presented in this chapter. The model includes policy formulation, implementation, and modification phases and emphasizes the interrelationships among the phases. These phases are subsequently treated in detail in Chapters 3, 4, and 5.

Chapter 6, "The Other Side of Policymaking," addresses the question of who the policymaking process affects, as well as the implications for them and for the process itself. Specific attention is given to the organizations that provide health care services or resources used in the production of these services as well as to the organizations and associations that represent the service and resource producers. Consideration is also given to the effect of policies on consumer groups and on employers. A common thread running through all of those affected by health policies is their dual concerns of discerning the impacts of policies and of influencing the policies that affect them. Both concerns are addressed in this chapter.

Chapter 7, "Synthesizing the Policymaking Process," introduces a more abstract model of the policymaking process to illustrate how closely intertwined policy formulation, implementation, and modification are in reality. In addition, three critical influences on health policymaking in the United States in the years immediately ahead are identified: the goals and objectives of health policy, about which we in the United States have had great difficulty in reaching consensus; the dynamics of the political marketplace, a most fascinating place in which participants pursue such self-interests as economic or political advantage as well as the public interest; and the painful fact that health policy decisions must eventually be made within the context of economic scarcity.

The book concludes with an appendix that lists chronologically the most important federal laws pertaining to health enacted in the United States. Aside from providing synopses of these laws, the chronology also reveals several important characteristics of the nation's health policies. For example, the list clearly shows that many health policies are but modifications of or amendments to previously enacted laws. Incrementalism has indeed prevailed in the development of American health policy. The list also shows that our approach to health policy mirrors the various determinants of health. There are policies to address the environments in which people live, their lifestyles, and their genetics, as well as extensive policies related to the nation's health care system.

I wish to acknowledge the contributions several people made to this book. Some of my colleagues at the University of Pittsburgh critiqued early drafts of the manuscript and were especially helpful in refining the model of the policymaking process presented in this book. George Board, Morton Coleman, Judith Lave, Ray Owen, Margaret Potter, Edmund Ricci, and Louis Tronzo generously provided helpful insights and suggestions. James Morone of Brown University, in his role as editor of the *Journal of Health Politics, Policy and Law*, encouraged me in the development of the book even as he rejected a manuscript on the topic of health policymaking as too long for his journal. John Parascandola, U.S. Public Health Service Historian, kindly reviewed the chronology of federal laws in the appendix of this book and made a number of helpful suggestions. John Fanning of the Office of Health Planning and Evaluation of the U.S. Department of Health and Human Services, also reviewed the chronology and helped me make the chronology more complete. Royall Tyler of the Australian National University in Canberra graciously permitted me to use his translation of a passage from the *Takasago* on the dedication page.

I also wish to acknowledge the contribution to my thinking about the process of policymaking made by two authors. John W. Kingdon's important book, *Agendas, Alternatives, and Public Policies*, has helped many people, including me, to better understand how public policies are made in the United States. Pamela A. Paul-Shaheen developed the first model of the policymaking process that I found complete enough to enthusiastically share with my students. It can be found in her article, "Overlooked Connections: Policy Development and Implementation in State-Local Relations," *Journal of Health Politics, Policy and Law* 45, no. 4 (Winter 1990): 833–56. My model of the policymaking process, like so much scholarship, draws on, adapts, and extends the work of others. The influence of both Kingdon and Paul-Shaheen can be clearly seen in my model of policymaking and is gratefully acknowledged here.

I appreciate the intellectual environment in which it has been my privilege to work for many years at the University of Pittsburgh. The efforts to establish and foster this environment by Chancellor Dennis O'Connor, by Senior Vice Chancellor for the Health Sciences Thomas Detre, and by the Dean of the Graduate School of Public Health, Don Mattison, are deeply appreciated.

I thank several people at Health Administration Press for their part in making this book possible. Sandra Crump, Tracy Flynn, Ed Kobrinski, and Kelly Sippell each contributed professional expertise and helpful support in the book's editing and production. Their work is much appreciated.

I thank Elly Poster and Lily Maskew, at the University of Pittsburgh, for doing onerous support work on this book effectively and cheerily.

Finally, I thank my family for their support and help in what I do. Brant, having just entered the world of young adulthood, gives me hope that his generation will do better with health policy, and a lot of other things, than mine. Courtland, on the brink of adolescence, is a constant source of wonderment and joy. It amazes and pleases me that one of his favorite places remains a stool beside my chair. I am especially grateful to my wife, Carolyn, to whom this book is dedicated, for encouraging this project and for her critiques of the book in progress. Her intelligence, style, and wisdom are among my greatest writing allies and they are deeply appreciated.

1

Health and Health Policy

$\mathbf{H}$ealth is extensively and tightly interwoven into the social and economic fabric of the United States. It plays a critically important role in the physical, psychological, and economic condition of the American people and of their society. Thus, health receives considerable attention from the nation's policymakers. This book is about the intricate public policymaking process they use to influence our pursuit of health. In this first chapter, some basic and underpinning definitions and concepts will be established. In the next chapter, a general model of the public policymaking process will be described. The various interconnected parts of the model will then be used as the means to organize subsequent chapters. Our exploration of the process through which health policy is established begins with some key definitions.

What Is Health?

Although it is important to every human being, there is no universally accepted definition of health. Health is routinely conceptualized by different people in both negative and positive terms and both narrowly and broadly. Negatively, health is viewed as the minimization, if not the absence, of some variable, as in the absence of infection or the shrinking of a tumor. At the extreme negative end of definitions, health is thought of as the absence of disease. Positively, health is viewed as a state in which some variable is maximized. For example, viewing health positively and broadly, the World Health Organization (1948) has defined health as the state of complete physical, mental, and social well-being, and not merely the absence of disease. This positive and broad definition of health describes an ideal state, not necessarily one that can be attained or, for that matter, fully measured.

Considering the definition of health is important because the way in which a society defines health reflects its values and how far it might be willing to go toward maximizing health among its members. A society that defines health in negative terms and narrowly, for instance, might choose to intervene only in life-threatening traumas and illnesses. Conversely, a society in which health is defined in positive terms and broadly might obligate itself to pursue a variety of significant interventions in pursuit of health for its members. As the United States has matured as a society, it has moved toward defining health in ever more positive and broader terms. One workable, contemporary definition of health holds that *health* is the maximization of the biological and clinical indicators of organ function and the maximization of physical, mental, and role functioning in everyday life (Brook and McGlynn 1991). This is a positive, and very broad, definition of health.

The consequences for a society that defines health positively and broadly are substantial. In contrast to focusing on treatment of illness or injury so as to minimize an undesired variable, it encourages society to seek proactive interventions aimed at many variables in the quest for health. The enormous range of possible targets for intervention is illustrated by the fact that health in human beings is determined by several synergistically related factors. Among these *health determinants*, perhaps none is more important than the physical, sociocultural, and economic environments in which people live (Blum 1983). In addition, health is strongly influenced by the lifestyles people lead and by heredity.

Health is also affected by the type, quality, and timing of health care services that people receive. *Health care services* are activities undertaken specifically to maintain or improve health or to prevent decrements of health. These services can be preventive, acute, chronic, restorative, or palliative in nature. The *health care system* is the resources (money, people, physical infrastructure, and technology) and the organizational configurations used to transform these resources into health care services. These definitions and considerations of health, health determinants, health care services, and the health care system should be kept in mind in considering policymaking. Ultimately, they help shape the purpose and focus of health policy.

What Is Health Policy?

In view of the desirability of health and the fundamental contribution of health care services to the physical and psychological condition of the citizenry, as well as the role that the quest for health plays in the nation's economy, it is not surprising that government, at all levels, is keenly interested in health affairs. This interest is reflected vividly in the diverse activities that occur within the expansive forum of public policymaking and in the resulting public policies that pertain to our pursuit of health, including policies affecting the provision and financing of health care services and production of the inputs to those services.

Public policies are authoritative decisions made in the legislative, executive, or judicial branches of government intended to direct or influence the actions, behaviors, or decisions of others. When public policies pertain to or influence our pursuit of health, they become *health policies*. Generally, health policies affect groups or classes of individuals (such as physicians, the poor, the elderly, or children) or types or categories of organizations (such as medical schools, health maintenance organizations, medical technology producers, employers, or nursing homes).

In the United States, health policies are made within a dynamic public policymaking process involving many interactive participants in several interconnected phases of activities. Federal, state, and local levels of government establish health policies. At any given time, the entire set of such policies made at any level of government can be said to form that level's *health policy*.

Policies made through the public policymaking process are distinguished from policies made in the private sector. It is beyond the scope of this book to discuss private sector health policies, such as decisions made by insurance companies about their product lines, pricing, and marketing or decisions made by the Joint Commission on Accreditation of Healthcare Organizations (JCAHO), a private accrediting organization, about what criteria to use in their reviews of organizations, as well as the processes through which such policies are made in the private sector. The focus here is restricted to the public policymaking process and the public sector health policies that result from this process. But there are indeed private sector health policies and they play a vitally important role in the health of Americans.

Forms of health policies

Health policy, especially at the national and state levels, is comprised of a very large set of decisions. Some of these decisions are codified in the statutory language of specific pieces of legislation. Others are the rules and regulations established in order to implement legislation or to operate government and its various programs. Still others are the judicial branch's decisions related to health. Examples of health policies include: the 1965 legislation that established the Medicare and Medicaid programs; an executive order regarding operation of federally funded family planning clinics; a court's decision that the merger of two hospitals violates federal antitrust laws; a state government's decisions about its procedures for licensing physicians; a county health department's decisions about its procedures for licensing restaurants; and a city government's enactment of an ordinance banning smoking in public places within the city. Thus, health policies may take any of several specific forms.

Statutes/Laws and programs

Statutes or *laws*, such as the statutory language contained in the 1983 Amendments to the Social Security Act (P.L. 98-21) that authorized the prospective payment system (PPS) for reimbursing hospitals for Medicare beneficiaries or the statutory language that defines which providers in a state can participate in the state's Medicaid program, are policies. Laws, when they are "more or less freestanding legislative enactments aimed to achieve specific objectives" (Brown 1992, 21), are sometimes called *programs*. The Medicare and Medicaid programs are examples. An example on a smaller scale is the Women, Infants, and Children (WIC) program, which is a federal initiative undertaken to improve health by reducing nutritional deficits for the beneficiaries of the program. Another example can be found in the certificate-of-need (CON) programs through which many states seek to influence capital expansion in their health care systems.

Rules/Regulations

Another form policies can take are the *rules* or *regulations* established to guide the implementation of laws and programs. Such rules, made in the executive branch of government by the organizations and agencies responsible for implementing laws and programs, and issued under the authority of law, are also policies. The rules associated with the implementation of complex statutes fill thousands of pages. Rulemaking, as an important activity in the larger policymaking process is covered in depth in Chapter 4.

Judicial decisions

Judicial decisions are another form of policies. For example, the Supreme Court's reversal in 1988 of the earlier decision of the United States Court of Appeals for the Ninth Circuit in the *Patrick v. Burget* case (a case involving the relationship between peer review of professional activities and antitrust liability) is a policy by our earlier definition because it is an authoritative decision that has the effect of directing or influencing the actions, behaviors, or decisions of others. As is often the case with judicial decisions, this one disrupted an established pattern of prior decisions and behaviors. Similarly, an opinion issued in 1992 by a U.S. Department of Health and Human Services administrative law judge that a hospital was in violation of the Rehabilitation Act Amendments of 1974

(P.L. 93-516) when it prohibited a HIV-positive staff pharmacist from preparing intravenous solutions is also a policy (Lumsdon 1992).

Macro policies

A fifth form health policies can take, but one that is only now emerging in the United States, is broad *macro policies*. Such policies "shape the health care system by constraining the flow of resources into it and setting limits on key players' freedom of action" (Brown 1992, 21). A good example of such a policy would be the imposition by the federal government of a global budget for the nation's health care system. While macro policies are new to the United States, most other advanced nations, Canada and Great Britain notably, have had such policies in place for their health care systems for decades.

Categories of health policies

The United States is a capitalist nation where the presumption is that private markets best determine the production and consumption of goods and services, including health services. While the volume and variety of existing health policies seem incongruous with the fact, government generally intrudes with policies only when private markets fail to achieve desired public objectives. The most credible arguments for policy intervention in the nation's domestic activities begin with the identification of situations in which markets are not functioning properly.

The health sector seems especially prone to situations in which markets do not function well (Congressional Budget Office 1991). Theoretically perfect (i.e., competitive) markets, which do not exist in reality, require certain conditions: that buyers and sellers have sufficient information to make informed decisions, that a large number of buyers and sellers participate, that more sellers can easily enter the market, that each seller's products or services are satisfactory substitutes for those of their competitors, and that the quantity of products or services available in the market does not swing the balance of power toward either buyers or sellers.

The markets for health services in the United States violate these underpinnings of competitive markets in a number of ways. The complexity of health services reduces the ability of consumers to make informed decisions without guidance from the sellers. The entry of sellers in health services markets is heavily regulated. And widespread insurance coverage affects the decisions of both buyers and sellers in these markets. These and other factors mean that the markets for health services do not function competitively, thus inviting policy intervention.

Furthermore, the potential for private markets, on their own, to fail to meet public objectives related to health is not limited to the production and consumption of health services. For example, markets might not stimulate the conduct of enough socially desirable medical research or the education of enough physicians or nurses without the stimulus of policies that subsidize certain costs. Energy producers might not be sufficiently concerned about air pollution if such concerns interfere with their profitability or competitive positions in the absence of policies that penalize polluting behaviors.

These and many other similar situations in which markets do not lead to desired outcomes provide the philosophical basis for the establishment of health policies. The nature of the problems they are intended to overcome or ameliorate help shape health policies in a direct way. Health policies fit, broadly, into allocative or regulatory categories, although there is considerable potential for overlap between the categories (Bice 1988; Williams and Torrens 1993).

Allocative policies

Allocative policies are designed to provide net benefits to some distinct group or class of individuals or organizations, at the expense of others, in order to ensure that public objectives are met. Such policies are in essence subsidies through which policymakers seek to alter demand for or supplies of particular goods and services or to guarantee access to goods and services for certain people. For example, on the basis that markets would undersupply the preparation of physicians without subsidies to medical schools, government has heavily subsidized the medical education system (e.g., P.L. 88-129, the Health Professions Education Act of 1963). On the basis that markets would undersupply hospitals in sparsley populated regions or low-income areas, government has subsidized the construction of hospitals (e.g., P.L. 79-725, the Hospital Survey and Construction Act of 1946).

Other subsidies have been used to ensure that certain people have access to health services. The most obvious examples of such policies are the Medicare and Medicaid programs.[1] But federal funding to support health services for Native Americans, veterans, and migrant farm workers and state funding for mental institutions are other examples of allocative policies intended to assist individuals in gaining access to needed services. Such subsidies as those inherent in much of the financial support for medical education, the Medicare program, the benefits of which are not based on the financial need of the recipients, and the exclusion from taxable income of employer-provided health insurance benefits indicate that poverty is not a necessary condition for the receipt of the subsidies available through allocative health policies.

Regulatory policies

Policies designed to influence the actions, behaviors, and decisions of others through directive (sometimes called command and control) techniques are regulatory policies.[2] As with allocative policies, the purpose of regulatory policies is to ensure that public objectives are met. There are five basic classes of regulatory policies: (1) market entry restrictions; (2) rate or price-setting controls on providers; (3) provider quality controls; and (4) market-preserving controls, all of which are variations of economic regulation; and (5) social regulation, which seeks to achieve such socially desired ends as safe workplaces, nondiscriminatory provision of health care, and reduction in the negative externalities (side-effects) that can be associated with the production or consumption of goods and services (Bice 1988; Williams and Torrens 1993). The regulatory activities of state and federal levels of government are discussed in more detail in Chapter 2 and, especially, in Chapter 4.

Whether public policies take the form of statutes or laws, programs, rules and regulations, judicial decisions, or macro policies, they are always established within the context of a complex public policymaking process. Both allocative and regulatory policies are made within the process, and the activities and mechanisms used to create both categories of policies are essentially identical. A comprehensive model of this process, which can apply to any level of government, is presented in Chapter 2. But before examining the model, it will be useful to consider the ways that health policies affect health. There is, in fact, a direct and crucially important connection between health policies and health.

The Impact of Health Policies on Health

Ideally, from government's perspective, the central purpose of health policy is to enhance health. Of course, it is possible for other purposes to be served by specific health policies; these could include economic advantages for certain individuals and organizations or the nation's general economic condition. But the defining purpose of health policy, so far as government is concerned, is to support the quest for health by the nation's citizenry.

Health policies, by definition, are intended to influence the actions, decisions, and behaviors of people in the domains of the environmental conditions under which people live; their lifestyles and personal behaviors; and through improvements in the availability, accessibility, and quality of their health care services. Thus, it is important to consider the role of health policy in the environmental conditions (including physical, sociocultural, and economic environments) under which people live; in the behavioral choices that people make; and in the health care system that serves them.

Health policies and the environment

Many Americans are routinely exposed to a variety of harmful agents in their environments. Exposure or potential exposure to asbestos, excessive noise, ionizing radiation, toxic chemicals, and many other dangerous agents are part of their everyday lives. Some of the exposure is to agents such as synthetic compounds that are introduced into the environment as by-products of technological growth and development. Some exposure is to wastes that result from the manufacture, use, and disposal of a vast range of products. And some of the exposure is to naturally occurring agents such as carcinogenic ultraviolet radiation from the sun or naturally occurring radon gas in the soil. Often, the hazardous effects of naturally occurring agents are exacerbated by their combination with agents introduced by human activities. For example, the widespread use of freon in air conditioning systems and of chlorofluorocarbons (CFCs) in aerosolized products has reduced the protective ozone layer in earth's upper atmosphere, allowing an increased level of ultraviolet radiation from the sun to strike the planet's inhabitants. Similarly, exposure to naturally occurring radon gas appears to act synergistically with cigarette smoke as a carcinogenic hazard.

The health effects of exposure to hazardous agents, no matter how they are introduced into or naturally occur in the environment, is increasingly well understood. Air, polluted by a number of agents, has a direct, measurable effect on such diseases as asthma, emphysema, lung cancer, and on the aggravation of cardiovascular disease. Asbestos, which can still be found in buildings constructed prior to the ban on its use, causes pulmonary disease. Lead-based paint, also still found in older buildings and especially concentrated in poorer urban communities, when ingested, causes permanent neurological defects in infants and young children.

In what he terms its "environmental tradition," Thompson (1981) points out that government has been involved in a variety of efforts to exorcise environmental health hazards. Examples of such efforts abound in a number of federal policies, including: the Clean Air Act of 1963, the Flammable Fabrics Act of 1967, the Occupational Health and Safety Act of 1970, the the Consumer Product Safety Act of 1972, the Noise Control Act of 1972, and the Safe Drinking Water Act of 1974.

In addition to their physical environments, the sociocultural and economic environments that people encounter also play important roles in their health and in their utilization of health care services. Chronic unemployment, changes in family structure, poverty, homelessness, substance abuse, violence, and despair affect health as surely as harmful viruses or carcinogens.

In spite of improvement over the past 30 years, people who live in poverty continue to experience worse health status than people who are more affluent. African-Americans, Hispanic-Americans, and Native Americans experience worse health status (i.e., more frequent and more severe health problems) than the white majority or other minorities (Butler 1988; Klerman 1992). Poor Americans, who are disproportionately African- and Hispanic-Americans, obtain their health care services in a different manner than the non-poor. Instead of receiving care that is more coordinated, continuing, and comprehensive, the poor are far more likely to receive a patchwork of services, provided for the most part by public hospitals and by local health departments. Poor people are more often treated episodically, with one provider intervening in one episode of illness but with someone else involved in the next episode.

The impact of economic conditions is especially dramatic for children. Poor children have double the rates of low birth weight and more than double the rates of conditions that limit school activity compared to other children (Starfield 1992). Poor children are more likely to become ill and to have more serious illnesses than other children because of their increased exposure to harmful environments, inadequate preventive services, and restricted access to all types of health care services.

The impact of the economic environment on health is not limited to the poor however. Increasingly, economic difficulties are affecting a wider circle of Americans in regard to health. Today the entire nation bends under the weight of intractable federal budget deficits (see Table 1.1). Coupled with growing international trade deficits, these massive budget deficits portend a frightening economic environment for the future, one that features a reduced standard of living for many people. Such a forecast contains a deadly one-two punch for the health of those

Table 1.1   The Federal Budget Outlook through the Year 2000 (in billions of dollars)

	1992	1993	1994	1995	1996	1997	1998	1999	2000
Revenues	$1,088	$1,162	$1,242	$1,323	$1,390	$1,455	$1,534	$1,612	$1,693
Outlays	1,402	1,493	1,511	1,567	1,644	1,745	1,845	1,962	2,093
Deficit	314	331	268	244	254	290	311	350	400

Source: U.S. Congressional Budget Office, *The Economic and Budget Outlook: An Update*, Washington, DC: U.S. Government Printing Office, 1992.

in poorer economic circumstances: worsening health status, accompanied by growing difficulty in obtaining resources to devote to health care services.

Economic constraints are only part of a larger set of difficulties that unevenly affect Americans in their quests for health. Living in an inner city or rural setting often increases the challenge of finding a suitable source of health care services because the availability of providers is not adequate in many of these locations. Lack of information or inadequate information about health and about health care services is a significant disadvantage—one compounded by language barriers, functional illiteracy, or marginal mental retardation. Cultural backgrounds and ties, especially among many Native Americans, Hispanics, and Asian immigrants, for all the support they can provide, sometimes also create a formidable barrier between people and the mainline health care system. Such barriers are often especially effective in inhibiting preventive care and prenatal care.

Health policies and human behavior and genetics

As Rene Dubos observed decades ago, "To ward off disease or recover health, men [as well as women and children] as a rule find it easier to depend on the healers than to attempt the more difficult task of living wisely" (1959, 110). The price of this attitude is partially reflected in Table 1.2, which shows the impact on mortality of conditions related to genetic, environmental, and behavioral causes.

Heart disease illustrates both the opportunity for improvement and the continuing threat to health of the diseases with genetic, environmental, and behavioral causes. The death rate from heart disease declined by 40 percent between 1970 and 1990. While aggressive early treatment of heart disease has played a role in reducing the death rate from this disease, better control of several established risk factors, including cigarette smoking, elevated blood pressure, elevated levels of cholesterol, and obesity, also helps explain much of this improvement. Yet, even with this impressive improvement, heart disease remains the most common cause of death and will continue to be an important cause for the foreseeable future. Clearly, more can be done to prevent this disease than has been or is likely to be done.

The outlook for cancer, which is a category of diseases in which genetic, environmental, and behavioral causes play important roles, is very bleak. It is estimated that about 30 percent of the people now living in the United States will develop cancer (American Cancer Society 1989). The death rate from cancer can be expected to continue to grow throughout the decade. Much of the growth is attributable to lung cancer, a type of

Table 1.2   Age-Adjusted Death Rates by Selected Causes: 1970, 1980, 1990 (rates per 100,000 population)

Cause of Death	1970	1980	1990
Major cardiovascular diseases	340.1	256.0	189.8
Diseases of heart	253.6	202.0	152.0
Cerebrovascular diseases	66.3	40.8	27.7
Malignancies	129.9	132.8	135.0
Of respiratory and intrathoracic organs	28.4	36.4	41.4
Of digestive organs and peritoneum	35.2	33.0	30.2
Of breast	12.6	12.5	12.7
Accidents and adverse effects	53.7	42.3	32.5
Pneumonia and influenza	22.1	12.9	14.0
Diabetes mellitus	14.1	10.1	11.7
Chronic liver disease and cirrhosis	14.7	12.2	8.6
Homicide and legal intervention	9.1	10.8	10.2
AIDS	0.0	0.0	15.4

Sources: U.S. Bureau of the Census, *Statistical Abstract of the United States: 1993*, 113th ed. Washington, DC: The Bureau, 1993. AIDS data from the Centers for Disease Control.

cancer that is strongly correlated with behaviors and environmental exposures. Brightening this bleak picture somewhat are potential developments in gene therapy as a new weapon in the battle against some cancers.

Deaths from violence (including accidents, homicides, and suicides), liver cirrhosis, and AIDS (acquired immunodeficiency syndrome), which emerged in the 1980s and became one of the top ten leading causes of death by 1990, are caused by human behaviors. Yet attempts to impose behavioral restrictions involving mandatory seatbelt use, motorcycle helmet use, moderation in alcohol use, or firearms control have met with limited public support and very limited success. Policymakers have been reluctant to impose penalties for behaviors that lead to illness and death or to provide overt rewards for the avoidance or modification of such behaviors. To date, health policy interventions in diseases that are behaviorally caused or exacerbated have favored increased funding for research into the behaviors or increased efforts to influence behavior through education. Venturing beyond these actions into the domains of individual choice and liberty rights has been carefully avoided.

Table 1.3 National Health Expenditures in the United States, 1980–2000

Item	1980	1990	1991	1992	1993	1995	2000
				Amount in Billions			
National health expenditures	$250.1	$666.2	$736.5	$819.9	$903.3	$1,101.9	$1,739.8
Private	145.0	383.6	413.0	443.5	482.2	573.0	859.9
Public	105.2	282.6	323.5	376.5	421.1	528.8	879.9
Federal	72.0	195.4	223.2	258.9	290.0	366.1	617.5
State and local	33.2	87.3	100.3	117.5	131.1	162.8	262.4
U.S. population*	235.1	259.6	262.2	264.7	267.2	272.0	283.0
Gross domestic product	$2,708	$5,514	$5,674	$5,909	$6,259	$7,069	$9,637
				Per Capita Amount			
National health expenditures	$1,064	$2,566	$2,809	$3,098	$3,380	$4,050	$6,148
Private	617	1,478	1,575	1,675	1,805	2,106	3,039
Public	447	1,089	1,234	1,422	1,576	1,944	3,109
Federal	306	753	852	978	1,085	1,346	2,182
State and local	141	336	383	444	490	598	927
				Percent Distribution			
National health expenditures	100.0	100.0	100.0	100.0	100.0	100.0	100.0
Private	58.0	57.6	56.1	54.1	53.4	52.0	49.4
Public	42.0	42.4	43.9	45.9	46.6	48.0	50.6
Federal	28.8	29.3	30.3	31.6	32.1	33.2	35.5
State and local	13.3	13.1	13.6	14.3	14.5	14.8	15.1
				Percent of Gross Domestic Product			
National health expenditures	9.2	12.1	13.0	13.9	14.4	15.6	18.1

*July 1 social security area population estimates in millions.

Adapted and reprinted with permission, as it appeared in Burner, S. T., Waldo, D. R., and McKusick, D. R. "National Health Expenditures Projections Through 2030," *Health Care Financing Review* 14, no. 1 (Fall 1992): 14.

Health policies and the health care system

The health care system (defined earlier as the resources and the organizational configurations used to transform them into health care services) in the United States is massive and complex. To provide a sense of its scope, some of the resources, which are the building blocks for the system, are described in this chapter. (Chapter 6 contains more information on the principal organizational configurations present in the system.) The scope and magnitude of the health care system is reflected in the enormous quantity and variety of resources—money, people, physical infrastructure, and technology—required to build and operate the system. Each type of resource is heavily affected by health policies.

Money

As shown in Table 1.3, national health expenditures are expected to continue their steep rise throughout the 1990s. These expenditures will very likely exceed $1.7 trillion by the year 2000 and consume approximately 18 percent of the nation's gross domestic product (GDP) (Burner, Waldo, and McKusick 1992). Already, spending on health is greater than for education and defense combined, and as health spending continues to consume a growing share of the nation's resources, fewer resources will be available for other uses. This pattern of extraordinary growth has been, and will continue to be, heavily influenced by a host of the nation's health policies.

As can be seen in Figure 1.1, almost 90 percent of health expenditures are for personal health services, with hospital care, physicians' services, and nursing home care comprising the bulk of these expenditures. Each of these types of services experienced dramatic inflation over the past three decades. Expenditures for hospital services increased at an average annual rate of 11.7 percent between 1960 and 1991; for physicians' services the average annual rate of increase for the same period was 11.2 percent, and for nursing home services it was 14.2 percent (U.S. Congress 1993, 24).

The increased personal health spending resulted from several factors. Three factors external to the health care system accounted for almost half of the increase. General price inflation made up the bulk of this, with population growth and demographic changes accounting for approximately 15 percent of the growth. The other half of the growth in personal health expenditures was a function of factors within the health care system: inflation in health care spending rose even faster than general inflation; the intensity of health services increased (i.e., technological advances made possible more treatments and tests); and per capita use of health care services increased.

Figure 1.1   Distribution of Health Expenditures, 1991, 1995, 2000

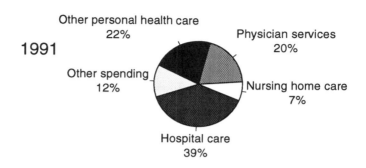

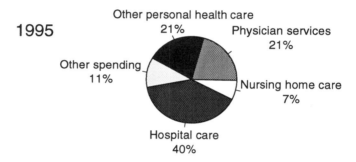

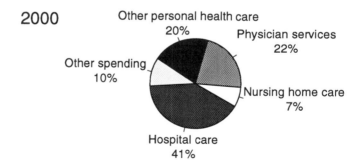

Notes: Other personal health care includes dental, other private professional services, home health care, drugs and other non-durable medical products, and vision products and other durable medical products. Other spending covers program administration and the net cost of private health insurance, government public health, and research and construction.

Adapted and reprinted with permission, as it appeared in Sonnefeld, S. T., Waldo, D. R., and McKusick, D. R. "Projections of National Health Expenditures Through the Year 2000," *Health Care Financing Review* 13, no. 1 (Fall 1991): 6.

The United States spends more on health than does any other country (Schieber, Poullier, and Greenwald 1992), in large part because of some significant variations in policies that affect health care services. For example, other countries have been far more likely to adopt policies such as global budgets for their health care systems, or to impose restrictive limitations on the supplies of health care services and on technology than has the United States (U.S. Congressional Budget Office 1991).

The implications of the level of health expenditures and the rate of increase in these expenditures over the past several decades are significant for both the public and private sectors. Summarizing a number of economic implications of these expenditures, the Congressional Budget Office has concluded that policymakers should be concerned about health costs for several reasons:

> First, health care markets are not truly competitive and therefore do not work very well. Because health care spending does not have to meet the usual market tests, health resources are not allocated efficiently. Too much money seems to be spent on procedures that have little value. At the same time, many people believe that too few resources are devoted to preventive care, such as immunizations. Such allocations may not reflect individual or social preferences, and many United States consumers do not believe that they are receiving their money's worth in health care.
>
> Second, rising health care costs have significantly reduced many people's access to medical care. An increasing number of people do not receive health insurance from their employers. Moreover, the costs of individual health policies have become prohibitively expensive for many. Without access to health insurance, studies have shown that these people receive reduced levels of medical care. Rising health care costs seem to be creating a dual system of medical treatment in the United States. Although most people enjoy access to the best and latest care in the world, an increasing number of people are shut out.
>
> Third, rising costs place significant burdens on workers. Rising health care costs have absorbed much of the growth of employees' real compensation over the past 20 years. Together with the slow growth of productivity, the rising costs of health insurance explain why workers' cash wages have hardly grown over the past two decades. The squeeze has meant that workers have less to spend on everything else. This situation has undoubtedly frustrated wage earners who have trouble making ends meet. These frustrations probably add to tensions between labor and management as well.
>
> Fourth, rising health care costs have most likely distorted the nation's labor market and made it less flexible. Because the costs of insurance are now so high, the availability of health insurance is becoming a more important factor in choosing a job. Moreover, rising costs may explain why large companies are eliminating positions for low-wage workers, such as janitors, and hiring independent contractors instead.

Fifth, rising health costs have also put substantial pressures on government budgets. Health programs are gobbling up a large portion of government resources and are threatening to crowd out other priorities, too. On the federal level, health spending is the only category of the budget, with the exception of net interest, that is rising as a share of gross domestic product (GDP). At the state level, increases in [health] costs will make it more difficult for states to fund other programs or provide tax relief. (Congressional Budget Office 1992, 8–9; Reprinted with permission of Congressional Budget Office Publications.)

People

The talents and abilities of a large and diverse workforce comprise another of the basic building blocks of the health care system. These human resources are directly affected by health policies. There are approximately 10.6 million health care workers in the United States today, reflecting more than a doubling of the number since 1970. They represent more than 11 percent of the nonagricultural workforce, and they represent the fastest growing group of American workers in the past decade (O'Neil 1993a).

The diversity of this workforce is reflected in the fact that the U.S. Department of Labor recognizes over 700 different job categories in the health care industry. There are about 600,000 active physicians, including about 28,000 who are osteopaths (D.O.s); 1.7 million registered nurses (RNs); 172,000 pharmacists; 140,000 active dentists; and more than 3 million allied health care workers in over 200 distinct disciplinary groups such as clinical laboratory technology, dental hygiene, dietetics, medical records administration, occupational therapy, physical therapy, radiologic technology, respiratory therapy, and speech-language pathology/audiology to name but a few (O'Neil 1993b).

Approximately half of the health care workforce is employed in hospitals, but the proportion who work in hospitals is declining as the organization and delivery of health care services becomes more decentralized and more often based in ambulatory settings (U.S. Department of Health and Human Services 1991). Demand for most health care disciplines is expected to continue to be strong through the remainder of this decade. The U.S. Department of Labor forecasts that demand for selected disciplines in the 1990s is expected to increase as follows: radiologic technicians by 66 percent, home health aides by 63 percent, physical therapists by 57 percent, surgical technicians by 56 percent, occupational therapists by 49 percent, and RNs by 39 percent (U.S. Department of Labor 1990).

The number of physicians has doubled in the past 30 years, largely in response to federal policies intended to increase the supply of physicians. For example, the Health Professions Educational Assistance Act of 1963 (P.L. 88-129) and its amendments of 1965, 1968, and 1971 helped to double the capacity of the medical schools in the United States by the early 1990s. However, the proportion of physicians who are primary care physicians (i.e., general practice, family practice, general internal medicine, and general pediatrics) has actually declined to about one-third. The decline is likely to continue during the 1990s (Rosenblatt 1992) and is of particular concern in view of the extensive efforts that have been made in the past two decades to increase the number and proportion of primary care physicians (Mick and Moscovice 1993).

Two-thirds of RNs work in the hospital setting, but nursing employment in nonhospital settings is growing rapidly, especially in health maintenance organizations (HMOs) and in home health agencies. As noted earlier, increased demand for nurses can be expected through the end of this decade and beyond. Demand will continue for nurses in their traditional patterns of practice, and increased demand for nurses in expanded primary care roles (e.g., nurse practitioners and nurse midwives), highly specialized care roles (e.g., clinical nurse specialists and nurse clinicians), and administrative roles can be expected. Projections are that a shortage of about 100,000–150,000 nurses per year will persist until early in the next century, and then grow more severe (O'Neil 1993b).

Physical infrastructure

Another building block of the health care system is the nation's investment in the "bricks and mortar" of physical facilities required to meet health care needs. Perhaps the most highly visible of these facilities are the nation's 6,700 hospitals. A hospital is "a health care institution which has an organized professional staff and medical staff and inpatient facilities, and which provides medical, nursing, and related services" (Slee and Slee 1991, 204). Various states establish specific criteria for the licensure of hospitals, often including the types of services that they must provide in order to qualify as a hospital.

There are about 33 million admissions to hospitals annually, and on any given day about 850,000 people are inpatients in the nation's hospitals. In addition, more than 350 million outpatient visits are made to these facilities annually. Hospitals vary dramatically in terms of size and scope of services, and there are a variety of ownership arrangements. There are 5,342 community, acute care hospitals, 930 specialty hospitals (e.g., psychiatric, rehabilitation, long-term care), and 334 federal hospitals open only to military personnel, veterans, or Native Americans. Of the community hospitals, nonprofit hospitals represent 59 percent, local government hospitals 27 percent, and for-profit hospitals 14 percent

(American Hospital Association 1992; De Lew, Greenberg, and Kinchen 1992).

Another important category of facilities where health care services are provided is generically referred to as nursing homes. A nursing home is "an institution which provides continuous nursing and other services to patients who are not acutely ill, but who need nursing and personal services as inpatients. A nursing home has permanent facilities and an organized professional staff" (Slee and Slee 1991, 298). This category of health care facilities is sometimes subdivided into skilled nursing facilities (SNFs), where on-site RN supervision is available for at least two nursing shifts per day and intermediate care facilities (ICFs) where on-site registered nurse supervision is available for only one nursing shift per day. An ICF that serves the mentally retarded is called an ICF/MR.

There are almost 16,000 nursing homes in the United States, with more than 1.6 million licensed beds (Marion Merrel Dow, Inc. 1991). Spending on nursing home care has risen dramatically in the past three decades, from less than $1 billion in 1960 to about $75 billion at present. Expenditures for nursing home care are expected to reach $147 billion by the year 2000 (Burner, Waldo, and McKusick 1992).

In addition to the services provided by hospitals and nursing homes, a huge and growing volume of health care services are provided to people on an ambulatory basis. The facilities used to provide these services comprise a large, and growing, part of the physical infrastructure of the health care system. Much ambulatory care is rendered in the private offices of the nation's physicians and dentists, including those associated with health maintenance organizations (HMOs). Increasingly, physicians have joined together in single- or multispecialty groups (three or more physicians formally associated to provide medical care, with shared offices, expenses, and income), often requiring large office complexes. There are also about 1,200 ambulatory surgery centers, 2,000 diagnostic imaging centers, and 3,000 medical laboratories independent of those in physicians' offices or hospitals (Rakich, Longest, and Darr 1992).

Technology

Broadly defined, *medical technology* includes "the drugs, devices, and medical and surgical procedures used in medical care, and the organizational and supportive systems within which such care is provided" (Banta, Behney, and Willems 1981, 5). In this inclusive definition, drugs and devices mean the biological, chemical, and physical artifacts and products used in medical care delivery; medical and surgical procedures mean the clinical activities of practitioners; and organizational and supportive systems mean the structural, managerial, and financial elements of medical care delivery.

The technological base of modern health care services is quite remarkable and must be viewed as one of the important building blocks of the health care system. The United States produces and consumes more and spends far more for medical technology than any other nation; it has provided technology with a uniquely favorable environment. Technology is much more widely and readily available to the citizens of the United States than to those in other nations (Rublee 1989). Funding for the research and development (R&D) that leads to new technology is provided by both the federal government and the private sector; although over the past decade the federal government's relative share of total R&D for health technology has declined, while private industry's share has increased (Luce 1993).

As this review of the resource base of the health care system affirms, this system is structured and sustained from building blocks that include vast sums of money, many different categories of people with specialized training, a massive investment in physical infrastructure, and a well-supported and growing technological base. In large measure, the scope and magnitude of this resource base reflects the history of the nation's health policies to date.

The impact of health policies on the health care system

There is abundant evidence that the American health care system has been developed under extraordinarily favorable public policies. For example, the nation has a long history of support for the development of medical technology through policies that directly support biomedical research and that encourage private investment in such research. Established in the early 1930s, the National Institutes of Health (NIH) started with a budget of about $10 million. Today, following exponential growth, the NIH annual budget is close to $10 billion. Encouraged by policies that permit firms to recoup their investments in research and development, private industry spends even more than the NIH on biomedical R&D (National Institutes of Health 1991).

Another important antecedent of today's health care system was enactment in 1946 of the Hospital Survey and Construction Act (P.L. 79-725). Congress, in support of expanded availability of health services and improved facilities, enacted this legislation, known as the Hill-Burton Act after its authors, to provide funds for hospital construction. This marked the beginning of a decades-long program of extensive federal developmental subsidies to increase the availability of health services. Much of the physical plant resources described earlier reflects this and other supportive policies.

Another crucially important part of the development of the health care system, again one supported by public policy, has been the expansion of health care insurance coverage. Beginning during World War II when wages were frozen, health insurance and other benefits in lieu of wages became very attractive features of the American workplace. Encouraged by policies that excluded these fringe benefits from income or Social Security taxes and by a Supreme Court ruling that employee benefits, including health insurance, could be legitimately included in the collective bargaining process, employer-provided health insurance benefits grew rapidly in the middle decades of the twentieth century (Health Insurance Association of America 1992). Beyond private-sector growth came the passage in 1965 of the Medicare and Medicaid legislation, providing more access to mainstream medical care for the aged and many of the poor through publically subsidized health insurance. With enactment of these programs, fully 85 percent of the American population had some form of health insurance.

Achievements of the health care system. Sustained and encouraged by these and other generous and supportive policies, the health care system in the United States has achieved some marvelous successes. Without attempting to be comprehensive, some of the major achievements include: diagnostic and therapeutic capabilities that are the most advanced in the world; biomedical research that has brought us to the brink of understanding disease at the molecular level and intervening in diseases at the genetic level (see Figure 1.2); the widespread availability of the latest technology and most sophisticated clinical facilities; and the provision of significant levels of choice for most citizens about who their physicians are and about when and where they obtain health care services. Yet, in spite of these achievements, there is a growing awareness that the health care system has some fundamental problems and that the health care services it delivers are neither as effectively nor as efficiently provided as they could be.

Problems of the health care system. As its central problem, the system has generated decades of rapidly escalating costs, costs that threaten the capacity of the nation to keep pace and that exacerbate the health care problems of those who lack adequate financial resources to access the system. The cost-escalation phenomenon is seen most clearly in international comparisons. As was noted earlier, the United States spends more on health care than any other nation. Furthermore, its rates of growth, whether in absolute dollar terms or as a proportion of GDP, have increased faster than spending in other countries (Schieber, Poullier, and Greenwald 1992). As to why this is the case, it has been observed that

Figure 1.2   Scientific and Technological Progress in Health Care

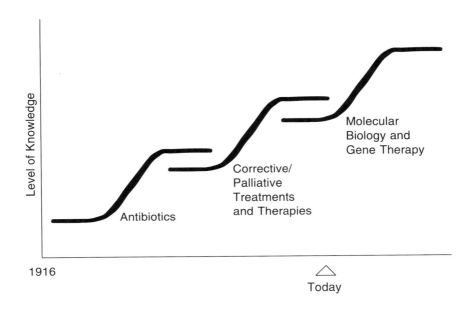

It is not that we are sicker or suffer from more expensive illnesses. All the Western countries are afflicted by nearly the same constellation of illnesses at roughly the same rates; for example, heart disease, cancer, and strokes are the major killers in all of them. It is not that we are aging disproportionately; all of the Western countries have aging populations. And it is not that we have unique, more expensive technology. The same technology is available in all the Western countries—although, to be sure, it is more widely disseminated in the United States. Nor is our health care better; by all the usual, albeit crude, measures of health outcome—for example, life expectancy, infant mortality, childhood immunization rate—the United States does somewhat worse than most Western countries. The only plausible explanation lies in the system—in the way health care is paid for and delivered in this country. Clearly, our system is peculiarly inefficient and inflationary. (Angell 1993, 1,778)

In addition to, and contributing to, the central cost problem, the system continues to create simultaneously excesses and shortages of various capabilities and facilities. We grossly underutilize primary care and preventive services, while overutilizing certain high-technology services.

One of the consequences of these problems is an inexorable pressure for change. As is so often the case in the United States, public pressure for change leads to new attempts to solve problems through changes in public policy. This phenomenon can be seen quite clearly in the political primacy of the health care reform movement in the early 1990s as reported by Starr (1992) and Enthoven (1993), among others.

The Citizenry and Health Policy

The citizenry of the United States is a remarkably diverse montage of people. While not capturing the full richness of their diversity, two demographic variables have significant importance for the health of the American people: the changing age structure of the population and its racial and ethnic diversity.

In 1990, about 32 million Americans were over the age of 65, and 13.5 million of them were over 75 years of age. By 2000, about 35.2 million will be over 65, with about 16.7 million of them over 75. By 2020, these numbers will increase to 52.7 million and 21 million (Burner, Waldo, and McKusick 1992). Older people consume relatively more health care services, and their health care needs differ from those of younger people. They also are more likely to consume long-term care services and community-based services intended to help them cope with various limitations in the activities of daily living.

Advancing age often means increased fragility and susceptibility to acute health problems such as injuries resulting from falls or infections and to chronic health problems such as emphysema or cirrhosis. Cardiovascular disease, cancer, diabetes, and osteoarthritis will remain serious health problems for elderly people well into the next century. Especially devastating can be the combination of acute and chronic health problems with cognitive impairments that occur with advancing age. Alzheimer's disease alone will affect 2.3 million Americans by the year 2000 (Centers for Disease Control 1990).

Although the view of the United States as a great melting pot of people and cultures was always more myth than reality, two groups now challenge this view in fundamental ways. African-Americans and especially Hispanic-Americans represent growing parts of the population. African-Americans have long faced fewer opportunities for education, employment, health care services, and for long and healthy lives compared to the numerically predominant European-Americans (Hacker 1992; Ayanian 1993). For some of the same reasons, and for a variety of others including language, geographic concentration, and cultural preferences, many Hispanic-Americans are also unlikely to become well-integrated into the dominant culture of the United States. These groups are presently underserved for health care services. Growth in their numbers exacerbates this problem, as does the fact that both groups are underrepresented in all of the health professions in the United States.

Although the population of the United States is diverse, including differences in health status, health care needs, and in access to the benefits of the health care system, the dominant culture reflects a rather homogeneous set of values that directly affects the nation's approach to health. The society, in general, places a high value on individual autonomy, self-determination, personal privacy, and maintains a widespread commitment to justice for all members of the society. Other characteristics of the core society that continue to influence health and health care include a deep-seated faith in the potential of technological rescue and, although it may be beginning to diminish ever so slightly, a longstanding obsession with prolonging life, with scant regard for the costs of doing so.

Finally, with particular relevance to the evolution of the nation's health policy, Americans have been extraordinarily reluctant to yield control of the health care system to government. In part, this reflects a unique feature of the American psyche. Perhaps Morone (1990, 1) has captured it best:

> At the heart of American politics lies a dread and a yearning. The dread is notorious. Americans fear public power as a threat to liberty. Their government is weak and fragmented, designed to prevent action more easily than to produce it. The yearning is an alternative faith in direct, communal democracy. Even after the loose collection of agrarian colonies had evolved into a dense industrial society, the urge remained: the people would, somehow, put aside their government and rule themselves directly.

Nowhere is this "dread and yearning" more visible than in regard to health and to health policy. Most of the human and physical resources utilized in the pursuit of health in the United States are under the control of the private sector. Even now, as the country experiments with a new level of government involvement in health care, the involvement focuses on finding ways to ensure broader access to health care services that will continue to be provided predominantly through the private sector and financed through the uniquely American mix of both public and private expenditures for health.

Conclusion

Health can be usefully conceptualized as the maximization of the biological and clinical indicators of organ function and the maximization of physical, mental, and role functioning in everyday life (Brook and McGlynn 1991). Thinking of health in this way emphasizes the need to address many variables if health is to be affected: the physical, sociocultural, and economic environments in which people live; their lifestyles, behaviors, and genetics; and the type, quality, and timing of health care services that people receive.

Health policies—which are authoritative decisions made within government that are intended to direct or influence the actions, behaviors, or decisions of others pertaining to health, health care services, or the health care system—are one of a developed society's principal means through which to exert an influence on health. The specific targets that health policies are intended to influence are the environmental conditions under which people live, their lifestyles and personal behaviors, and the availability, accessibility, and quality of their health care services.

No matter what the specific intent or target of policies, no matter what their form, health policies are made through a rather well-understood, although complex, process. The process is described in the next chapter, and details are provided in subsequent chapters.

Notes

1. Medicare is the principal social health insurance program in the United States. Enacted into law as Title XVIII of the Social Security Act (P.L. 89-97) on 30 July 1965, Medicare is a federally administered program and the nation's single largest health insurer. It covers 13 percent of the population for a variety of hospital, physician, and other health care services, including virtually all of those over the age of 65 as well as disabled individuals who are entitled to Social Security benefits and people with end-stage renal disease (Board of Trustees of the Federal Hospital Insurance Trust Fund 1992).

   The Medicare program includes two parts. Part A covers inpatient hospital care, very limited nursing home services, and some home health services and is earned through payment of a payroll tax during one's working years. In 1993, the tax was 1.45 percent of earnings for both the employer and the employee, for a total of 2.9 percent of annual income. Part B covers physician services, physician-ordered supplies and equipment, and certain ambulatory services such as hospital outpatient visits. Part B is voluntary, although about 97 percent of Part A beneficiaries choose to enroll in Part B. Part B of Medicare is paid for by a combination of enrollee monthly premiums ($41.10 in 1994) that cover about 25 percent of the costs and by general federal revenues that pay for about 75 percent of the costs. Since Medicare covered only 50 percent of the total health care expenses of elderly people, more than 75 percent of them purchased supplemental, or Medigap, health insurance plans in 1993 (Jensen 1993).

In essence, the Medicare program operates as an intergenerational transfer program in that taxes from working people are used to provide services to elderly beneficiaries. The inherent weakness in this approach to financing the program lies in the fact that while there were 5 workers for each beneficiary at the program's inception, there will be only 3 workers per beneficiary in 2000, and only 1.9 by 2040 (U.S. Congress 1991).

Medicaid, enacted along with Medicare, as Title XIX of the Social Security Act (P.L. 89-97), became an important part of the existing federal-state social welfare structure. It was intended to provide health insurance coverage for preventive, acute, and long-term care for some of the nation's poorer citizens. This program covers about 25 million people, or 10 percent of the population. In this program, the federal government provides a subsidy to the states (50 to 83 percent of the program's total costs depending on the per capita income in the state). In return for the subsidy, the states administer their Medicaid programs, but do so under broad federal guidelines regarding the scope of services to be covered, the level of payments to health care services providers, and eligibility requirements for coverage under the program.

Medicaid is public welfare; there is no entitlement as with Medicare and recipients must prove their eligibility in accordance with provisions of the program. Generally, eligibility requirements include being poor *and* aged, blind, disabled, pregnant, or the parent of a dependent child. Mothers and their dependent children comprise about 68 percent of those who receive Medicaid benefits, the elderly 13 percent (the improvished elderly receive this coverage in addition to Medicare benefits), the blind and disabled 15 percent, and others 4 percent (De Lew, Greenberg, and Kinchen 1992). Although eligibility criteria vary considerably from state to state, across the entire country only about 60 percent of the people who fall below the federal poverty line are covered by Medicaid (Swartz 1988). One of the ethically troubling aspects of this program results from the fact that since Medicaid covers long-term nursing home care, many middle-class elderly make themselves eligible for the program by transferring their assets to their children and exhausting their incomes on nursing home costs.

Medicaid is the fastest-growing component of most state budgets, a fact that has led many states to seek to reduce the growth of their Medicaid expenditures. States have followed various strategies to reduce these expenditures, including stringent preadmission screening for hospital care; limiting the number of hospital days available for program participants; reducing the amount of payment to health care service providers, often to a point below their costs of producing the services; increasing the copayment requirements for optional services; raising the eligibility standards, thereby reducing the number of people covered by the program; and limiting the range of services covered by the program.

2. In a variety of ways, government, at both federal and state levels, regulates certain of the actions, behaviors, and decisions of individuals and organizations. In part, they do this in the pursuit of certain public objectives related to health. (See, for example, Bice 1988; Williams and Torrens 1993.) There are several classes of such regulations.

   Entry-restricting regulations include those through which individual professionals such as physicians, dentists, and nurses, or organizations such as hospitals and nursing homes are licensed. Licensing is a state function, granted to them under the police powers granted to the states in the Constitution. Ostensibly, controls on the entry of providers into health care services markets have often been supported on the grounds that such controls help ensure quality and protect consumers from inadequately educated people or unsafe organizations. But market entry controls also serve to reduce the number of competitors in a market, thus policies that restrict the entry of competitors are usually favored by the providers who are already in a particular market. In addition to licensure regulations, state-operated certificate-of-need programs, through which approval for new projects by health care providers must be obtained from the state before the projects can be developed, are market entry–restricting regulation.

   Another class of regulations consists of those used to control the prices providers can charge for their services or the rates at which they are reimbursed. A common example of *price regulation* is government's control of the retail prices charged by public utilities, such as those that sell natural gas or electricity. Although it is not classified as a public utility, the health care industry is also subject to certain price regulations. For example, in an effort to help restrain inflation, the Nixon administration established the Economic Stabilization Program of 1971 through which wage and price controls were imposed on the health care industry (Ginsburg 1976). Currently, several states have established and continue to operate hospital cost- and rate-setting commissions (Eby and Cohodes 1985). Rate regulation with enormous impact is the federal government's control of the rates at which it reimburses hospitals for care provided to Medicare patients under the prospective payment system of reimbursement (Rowland 1991) and its establishment of a fee schedule for reimbursing physicians who care for Medicare patients (Ginsburg and Lee 1991).

   A third class of regulations are those intended to ensure that health care services providers adhere to acceptable levels of quality in the services they provide and that suppliers of health care products (e.g., imaging equipment or pharmaceuticals) meet safety and efficacy standards. The conceptual justification for such *quality control* regulatory intervention in the health care system rests on the view that consumers lack adequate information to judge quality. Thus, the Food and Drug Administration is charged to ensure that new pharmaceuticals meet safety and efficacy standards (Gelijns and Halm 1991). The federal government has established an elaborate system of peer review organizations (PROs) to evaluate the quality and appropriateness of care rendered to Medicare beneficiaries (Palmer, Donabedian, and Povar

1991). The Nuclear Regulatory Commission (NRC) enforces provisions of the Atomic Energy Act of 1954 and regulates and licenses the nuclear industry. In doing this, the NRC regulates hazards arising from the storage, handling, and transportation/disposal of nuclear materials, including those involved in the health care system.

In spite of the philosophical preference for having private markets determine the production and consumption of goods and services in the United States, including health care services, the reality is that such markets do not function perfectly. Indeed, they have major flaws in regard to health care services (U.S. Congressional Budget Office 1991). As a result, government intervenes in these markets by establishing and enforcing rules of conduct for market participants. These rules of conduct form a fourth class of regulation, *market-preserving controls*. This regulation takes the form of laws and judicial decisions that govern contracts and others that define and are used to punish antitrust violations. Antitrust laws are intended to maintain conditions that permit markets to work well and fairly. The laws governing contracts are intended to ensure that the economic exchanges that occur within markets follow predictable patterns. The U.S. Department of Justice and Federal Trade Commission enforce the Sherman Antitrust Act (1890) and the Clayton Act (1914) and their numerous amendments intended to prohibit anticompetitive practices.

The United States is entering a new era in regard to market-preserving regulations in the health care industry as it moves toward managed competition as a central element of its health policy (Enthoven 1993). As Bice (1988, 378) has pointed out, "While antitrust and other market-preserving laws are, technically speaking, regulatory devices, they are essentially passive, being invoked only when violated." Managed competition, which is a strategy to stimulate the development of vertically integrated networks of health care services providers and have them compete with each other for large pools of insured people within a framework that encourages cost-conscious decision making by consumers (Starr 1992; Starr and Zelman 1993), will likely require the elaboration of much more activist regulations if it is to work well. Already, for example, the regulations thought necessary to "manage" the competition in this market include the specification of benefit packages, changes in the tax treatment of employer-provided health insurance, and new and less restrictive policies governing eligibility for and transportability of health insurance coverage. In this context, existing antitrust laws are viewed by many as prohibiting the formation of new relationships and alliances among providers that will be needed to fully implement the concept of vertically integrated provider networks. Interestingly, the phrase managed competition, with the inclusion of the action oriented word, "managed," denotes a more activist or intrusive approach to the workings of the market for health care services.

The four classes of regulations outlined above are all variations of economic regulation. There is a fifth class that is termed *social regulation*. The primary intent of this class of regulations is to achieve such socially desirable outcomes as workplace safety and fair employment practices and to reduce such socially undesirable outcomes as environmental pollution or the spread of sexually transmitted diseases. Social regulation usually has economic impact, but the impact is secondary to the primary purposes of these regulations. Federal and state laws pertaining to environmental protection, disposal of medical wastes, childhood immunization requirements, and the mandatory reporting of communicable diseases are but a few obvious examples of social regulations. The Occupational Safety and Health Administration enforces provisions of the Occupational Safety and Health Act (1970) to help safeguard workplaces. The Equal Employment Opportunity Commission (EEOC) enforces the Equal Pay Act of 1963, Title VII of the Civil Rights Act of 1964, and Age Discrimination in Employment Act of 1967, among other laws, and investigates complaints about the treatment of employees by employers.

References

American Cancer Society. *Cancer Facts and Figures.* Atlanta, GA: American Cancer Society, 1989.

American Hospital Association. *Hospital Statistics, 1992–1993.* Chicago: The Association, 1992.

Angell, M. "How Much Will Health Care Reform Cost?" *New England Journal of Medicine* 328, no. 24 (17 June 1993): 1778–79.

Ayanian, J. Z. "Heart Disease in Black and White." *New England Journal of Medicine* 329, no. 9 (26 August 1993): 656-58.

Banta, H. D., C. J. Behney, and J. S. Willems. *Toward Rational Technology in Medicine.* New York: Springer Publishing Company, 1981.

Bice, T. W. "Health Services Planning and Regulation." In *Introduction to Health Services,* 3d ed., edited by S. J. Williams and P. R. Torrens, 373–405. New York: John Wiley & Sons, 1988.

Blum, H. K. *Expanding Health Care Horizons: From A General Systems Concept of Health to a National Health Policy,* 2d ed. Oakland, CA: Third Party Publishing Company, 1983.

Board of Trustees of the Federal Hospital Insurance Trust Fund. *1992 Annual Report of the Board of Trustees of the Federal Hospital Insurance Trust Fund.* Washington, DC: The Board, 1992.

Brook, R. H., and E. A. McGlynn. "Maintaining Quality of Care." In *Health Services Research: Key to Health Policy,* edited by E. Ginzberg, 784–817. Cambridge, MA: Harvard University Press, 1991.

Brown, L. D. "Political Evolution of Federal Health Care Regulation." *Health Affairs* 11, no. 4 (Winter 1992): 17–37.

Burner, S. T., D. R. Waldo, and D. R. McKusick. "National Health Expenditures Projections Through 2030." *Health Care Financing Review* 14, no. 1 (Fall 1992): 1–29.

Butler, P. A. *Too Poor To Be Sick: Access to Medical Care for the Uninsured.* Washington, DC: American Public Health Association, 1988.

Centers for Disease Control. *Morbidity and Mortality Weekly Report*, Vol. 39, No. 7. Atlanta, GA: Centers for Disease Control, 1990.

De Lew, N., G. Greenberg, and K. Kinchen. "A Layman's Guide to the U.S. Health Care System." *Health Care Financing Review* 14, no. 1 (Fall 1992): 151–69.

Dubos, R. *The Mirage of Health*. New York: Harper, 1959.

Eby, C. L., and D. R. Cohodes. "What Do We Know about Rate Setting?" *Journal of Health Politics, Policy and Law* 10, no. 2 (Summer 1985): 299–327.

Enthoven, A. C. "The History and Principles of Managed Competition." *Health Affairs* 12 (Supplement 1993): 24–48.

Gelijns, A. C., and E. A. Halm, eds. *The Changing Economics of Medical Technology*. Washington, DC: National Academy Press, 1991.

Ginsburg, P. B. "Inflation and the Economic Stabilization Program." In *Health: A Victim or Cause of Inflation?* edited by M. Zubkoff, 31–51. New York: Prodist-Milbank Memorial Fund, 1976.

Ginsburg, P. B., and P. R. Lee. "Physician Payment." In *Health Services Research: Key to Health Policy*, edited by E. Ginzberg, 69–92. Cambridge, MA: Harvard University Press, 1991.

Hacker, A. *Two Nations: Black and White, Separate, Hostile, Unequal*. New York: Macmillan, 1992.

Hamilton/KSA. *The Health Care Provider of the Future*. Fairfax, VA: Hamilton/KSA, 1992.

Health Insurance Association of America. *Source Book of Health Insurance Data*. Washington, DC: The Association, 1992.

Jensen, D. "Elderly Out-of-Pocket Health Care Expenditures, Part I: Sources of Liabilities." *Public Policy Institute of AARP Issue Brief* no. 16 (April 1993): 1–13.

Klerman, L. V. "Nonfinancial Barriers to the Receipt of Medical Care." *The Future of Children* 2, no. 2 (Winter 1992): 171–85.

Luce, B. R. "Medical Technology and Its Assessment." In *Introduction to Health Services*, 4th ed., edited by S. J. Williams and P. R. Torrens, 245–68. Albany, NY: Delmar Publishers, Inc., 1993.

Lumsdon, K. "HIV-Positive Health Care Workers Pose Legal, Safety Challenges for Hospitals." *Hospitals* 66, no. 18 (20 September 1992): 24–32.

Marion Merrel Dow, Inc. *Marion Merrel Dow Managed Care Digest: Long Term Care Edition* (pamphlet). Kansas City, MO: Marion Merrel Dow, Inc., 1991.

Mick, S. S., and I. Moscovice. "Health Care Professionals." In *Introduction to Health Services*, 4th ed., edited by S. J. Williams and P. R. Torrens, 269–96. Albany, NY: Delmar Publishers Inc., 1993.

Morone, J. A. *The Democratic Wish: Popular Participation and the Limits of American Government*. New York: Basic Books, 1990.

National Institutes of Health. *NIH Data Book*. Washington, DC: National Institutes of Health, 1991.

O'Neil, E. H. "Academic Health Centers Must Begin Reforms Now." *The Chronicle of Higher Education* (8 September 1993a): A48.

———. *Health Professions Education for the Future: Schools in Service to the Nation*. San Francisco, CA: Pew Health Professions Commission, 1993b.

Palmer, R. H., A. Donabedian, and G. J. Povar. *Striving for Quality in Health Care: An Inquiry into Policy and Practice.* Ann Arbor, MI: Health Administration Press, 1991.

Rakich, J. S., B. B. Longest, Jr., and K. Darr. *Managing Health Services Organizations,* 3d ed. Baltimore, MD: Health Professions Press, 1992.

Rowland, D. "Financing Health Care for Elderly Americans." In *Health Services Research: Key to Health Policy,* edited by E. Ginzberg, 127-60. Cambridge, MA: Harvard University Press, 1991.

Rosenblatt, R. A. "Specialists or Generalists: On Whom Should We Base the American Health Care System?" *Journal of the American Medical Association* 267, no. 12 (25 March 1992): 1665–67.

Rublee, D. A. "Medical Technology in Canada, Germany and the United States." *Health Affairs* 8, no. 3 (Fall 1989): 180.

Schieber, G. J., J. P. Poullier, and L. M. Greenwald. "U.S. Health Expenditure Performance: An International Comparison and Data Update." *Health Care Financing Review* 13, no. 4 (Summer 1992): 1–87.

Slee, V. N., and D. A. Slee. *Health Care Terms,* 2d ed. St. Paul, MN: Tringa Press, 1991.

Sonnefeld, S. T., D. R. Waldo, J. A. Lemieux, and D. R. McKusick. "Projections of National Health Expenditures Through the Year 2000." *Health Care Financing Review* 13, no. 1 (Fall 1991): 1–27.

Starfield, B. "Child and Adolescent Health Status Measures." *The Future of Children* 2, no. 2 (Winter 1992): 25–39.

Starr, P. *The Logic of Health-Care Reform: Transforming American Medicine for the Better.* Knoxville, TN: The Grand Rounds Press, 1992.

Starr, P., and W. A. Zelman. "Bridge to Compromise: Competition Under a Budget." *Health Affairs* 12 (Supplement 1993): 7–23.

Swartz, K. "How the Overlap Between the Poverty and Medicaid Populations Changed Between 1979 and 1983, or Lessons for the Next Recession." *Journal of Human Resources* 24, no. 2 (1988): 319–30.

Thompson, F. J. *Health Policy and the Bureaucracy: Politics and Implementation.* Cambridge: Massachusetts Institute of Technology Press, 1981.

U.S. Congress. House Committee on Ways and Means. *Health Care Resource Book.* Washington, DC: U.S. Government Printing Office, 1993.

———. *Overview of Entitlement Programs, 1991 Green Book.* Washington, DC: U.S. Government Printing Office, 1991.

U.S. Congressional Budget Office. *Economic Implications of Rising Health Care Costs.* Washington, DC: U.S. Government Printing Office, 1992.

———. *Rising Health Care Costs: Causes, Implications, and Strategies.* Washington, DC: U.S. Government Printing Office, 1991.

U.S. Department of Commerce. "U.S. Industrial Outlook 1993." Washington, DC: U.S. Government Printing Office, 1993.

U.S. Department of Health and Human Services. National Center for Health Statistics, Public Health Service. *Health United States, 1990.* Washington, DC: U.S. Government Printing Office, 1991.

U.S. Department of Labor. *Occupational Outlook.* Washington, DC: U.S. Government Printing Office, 1990.

Williams, S. J., and P. R. Torrens. "Influencing, Regulating, and Monitoring the Health Care System." In *Introduction to Health Services*, 4th ed., edited by S. J. Williams and P. R. Torrens, 377–96. Albany, NY: Delmar Publishers Inc., 1993.

World Health Organization. "Constitution of the World Health Organization, 1948." In *Basic Documents*, 15th ed. Geneva, Switzerland: World Health Organization, 1948.

Figure 2.1 A Model of the Public Policymaking Process in the United States

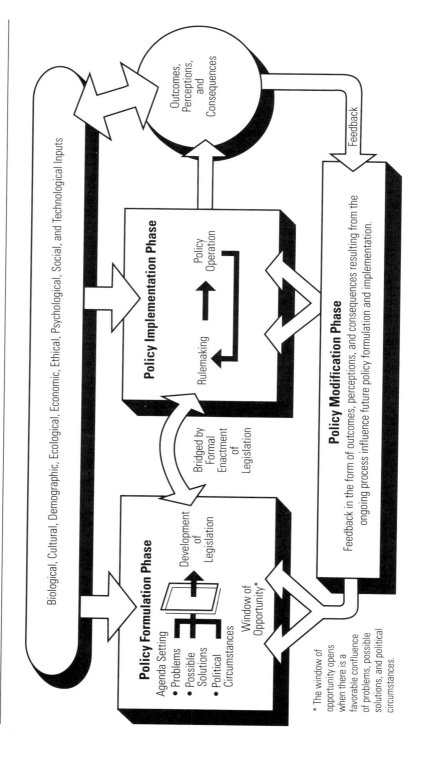

2

A Model of Public
Policymaking for Health

Whether public policies take the form of statutes or laws, programs, rules and regulations, judicial decisions, or macro policies, they are made through a well-established, although very complex, process. Both allocative and regulatory policies are made through the process, with the activities and mechanisms used to establish both categories of policies being essentially the same. A model of this process (see Figure 2.1), which can apply to any level of government, is presented in this chapter. We will apply this process model to making health policies, but it is also relevant to making public policies in other domains such as education, defense, and welfare.

It is a matter of convenience and convention for examination to separate the process of policymaking in one domain, such as health, from other related ones. In reality, the policymaking process in the United States rarely is so neat as to permit close examination of one domain without consideration of others. For example, it is impossible, as a practical matter, to consider health policy aside from its relationship to tax policy: "Government policy toward health care can never be separated from financing or tax issues, or from alternative uses and expenditures to which tax dollars might be devoted. In many discussions, health policy is treated as isolated from tax policy. Inevitably and irreducibly, however, they are two sides of the same accounting ledger" (Steuerle as quoted in Pear 1993a, E4).

A portion of the model on the facing page is influenced by and reprinted with permission by Duke University Press from P. A. Paul-Shaheen, "Overlooked Connections: Policy Development and Implementation in State-Local Relations." *Journal of Health Policy, Politics and Law* 15, no. 4 (Winter 1990). © Duke University Press, 1990. The conceptualization of a "window of opportunity" separating agenda setting from legislation development in policymaking can be traced to J. W. Kingdon in *Agendas, Alternatives, and Public Policies*, Boston: Little, Brown & Company, 1984.

Before examining the model of the policymaking process, the inter-connected components of which will form the outline for the remaining chapters in the book, it will be useful to first consider the political con-text—or political market—within which health policymaking occurs.

The Political Market for Health Policies

An understanding of the political market for health policies in the United States is largely based on a knowledge of the operation of traditional eco-nomic markets. Economic markets and political markets share a number of common features. Many kinds of goods and services, including those used in the pursuit of health, are bought and sold in the context of eco-nomic markets. In these markets, willing buyers and willing sellers enter into economic exchanges involving something of value to both parties. One party demands and the other supplies. By dealing with each other through market transactions, individuals and organizations buy needed resources and sell their outputs.

Since people are calculative regarding their relative rewards and costs incurred in exchanges, they often rely on contracts that, even if only implicit, govern most market transactions by defining the parameters of the exchanges between the participating parties. Contracts, as support-ing devices for economic market transactions, are often negotiated agree-ments between parties for the exchange of future performance. As such, contracts can rest simply on the faith and belief that each party will per-form as agreed or, more rigorously, on specific terms that can be evalu-ated by third parties and that can serve as the basis for penalties to be assessed if performance by parties to an agreement is not satisfactory. Thus, a key element in the effective operation of economic markets is the ability to negotiate acceptable agreements among buyers and sellers (Longest 1990).

Negotiation (or bargaining) involves two or more parties attempt-ing to settle what each shall give and take (or perform and receive) in an economic transaction between them. As we will see, this feature of eco-nomic markets has a parallel in the operation of political markets. In the interactions that take place in a negotiation in an economic market, the parties attempt to agree on a mutually acceptable outcome in a situation where their preferences for outcomes are usually negatively related. In-deed, if the preferences for outcomes are positively related, an agreement or contract can be reached almost automatically.

More typically, among parties to a negotiation, there are at least two types of issues that must be resolved through the negotiations. One type is the division of resources, the so-called "tangibles" of the negotia-tion, such as who will receive how much money, goods, or services in exchange for what considerations. Another type is the resolution of the psychological dynamics and the satisfaction of personal motivations of the parties in the negotiations. These issues are the so-called "intangibles" of the negotiation and can include such things as appearing to win or lose, to compete effectively, or to cooperate fairly.

Negotiations in economic exchange situations usually follow one of two strategic approaches—*cooperative* (win/win) or *competitive* (win/ lose) strategies. The choice of the negotiating strategy best utilized in any particular situation is a function of the interaction of several variables. Optimal conditions for the use of cooperative negotiating strategies are:

- The tangible goals of both negotiators are to attain a specific settlement that is fair and reasonable.
- There are sufficient resources available in the environment for both sides to attain their tangible goals, more resources can be attained, or the problem can be redefined so that both sides can actually "win."
- Each side believes (perceives) that it is possible for both of them to attain their goals through the negotiation process.
- The intangible goals of both negotiators are to establish a cooperative relationship and work together toward a settlement that maximizes their joint outcomes.

In contrast, the optimal conditions for the use of competitive negotiating strategies are:

- The tangible goals of both negotiators are to attain a specific settlement or to get as much as they possibly can.
- There are insufficient resources available for both sides to attain their goals, or their desires to get as much as possible makes it impossible for one or both parties to actually attain their goal(s).
- Both sides perceive that it is impossible for both of them to attain their goals.
- The intangible goals of both sides are to beat the other, keep the other from attaining his or her goals, humiliate the other, or refuse (for various reasons) to make concessions in one's own negotiating position. (Greenberger et al. 1988, 129)

The operation of political markets

Political markets for health policies operate much as do traditional economic markets, although there are certainly some key differences. The most fundamental difference is that in economic markets consumers express their preferences by spending their own money. That is, in economic markets consumers reap the benefits of their choices, and they also directly bear the costs of their choices. In political markets, on the other hand, the linkage between who receives benefits and who bears costs is not so direct.

Other characteristics that differentiate political markets from economic markets include the following:

> In private markets individuals make separate decisions on each item they purchase. They do not have to choose between sets of purchases, such as between one package that might include a particular brand of car, a certain size house in a particular neighborhood, several suits, and a certain quantity of food. Yet in political markets their choices are between two sets of votes by competing legislators on a wide variety of issues. While individual voters may agree or disagree on parts of the package, they cannot register a vote on each issue, as they do in economic markets.
>
> Voting participation rates differ by age group. The young and future generations do not vote, and yet policies are enacted that impose costs on them. Future generations depend on current generations and voters to protect their interests. However, as has been the case many times, such as with respect to the federal deficit and Social Security, their interests have been sacrificed to current voters.
>
> Legislators use different decision criteria than those used in the private sector. A firm or an individual making an investment considers both the benefits and the costs of that investment. Even though a project may offer very large benefits, profitability cannot be established unless its costs are also considered. Legislators, however, have a different time horizon, which not only affects the emphasis they place on costs and benefits but also on when each is incurred. Since members of the House of Representatives run for reelection every two years, they are likely to favor programs that provide immediate benefits (presumably just before the election) while delaying the costs until after the election or years later. Further, from the legislator's perspective, the program does not even have to meet the criterion that the benefits exceed its costs, only that the immediate benefits exceed any immediate costs. Future legislators can worry about future costs. (Feldstein 1988, 237–38)

Policies, which we have defined as authoritative decisions made in the legislative, executive, or judicial branches of government that are intended to direct or influence the actions, behaviors, or decisions of others, are among the commodities valued in the political marketplace (Marmor and Christianson 1982). Both those who "supply" policies and those individuals or groups who "demand" or "consume" policies recognize the innate value of policies; in political markets, both suppliers and demanders stand to reap benefits or incur costs because of policies.

The demanders of health policies

Viewing political markets as operating similarly to economic markets—that is, as markets in which something of value is exchanged between suppliers and demanders, and where policies are a valued commodity—permits policies to be viewed as means of satisfying demanders' wants and needs in the same way that private goods and services serve to satisfy demanders (usually called consumers) in private economic markets. In private markets, demanders seek goods and services that satisfy them. In political markets, demanders specifically seek policies that satisfy them. In both markets, suppliers provide the other side of the exchange equation.

Broadly, the demanders of health policies can include the entire citizenry. Conceptually at least, citizen-demanders can consider possible policies, including the impact of the policies on themselves and the people and things they care about. Based on their assessment, the citizen-demanders can select and support policymakers who they believe are most likely to help produce the favored policies and/or seek to influence policymakers to encourage them to help provide the desired policies. Influence by the citizen-demanders can be exerted through the power of the vote, campaign contributions, volunteered time to work in a campaign, or the provision of anything of value to the policymaker.

There is, however, a basic and very limiting problem with this conceptualization of citizen-demanders. For almost all individuals, the cost of such direct participation in the policymaking process is quite high. If they are to effectively participate, individuals must acquire substantial amounts of information about many policy options. This effort usually involves time and money, often in considerable amounts. Beyond this, individual participants often must be prepared to expend additional resources, again money and time, in support of achieving desired policies. Since most health policies do not provide significant, or in some cases even noticeable, benefits to most individuals, the high costs of participation generally mean that individual citizen-demanders participate in the political markets for policies to a very limited degree, at least as individuals.

The most effective demanders of policies, in view of the limited role of individuals, are the well-organized interest groups. (More is said about the structure and functions of interest groups in Chapter 3, and about the role of organizations in relation to policies in Chapter 6.) By combining and concentrating the resources of members, whether they be individuals such as physicians in the American Medical Association (AMA) or older citizens allied in the American Association for Retired Persons (AARP), or organizations such as hospitals in the American

Hospital Association (AHA) or the member companies in the Pharmaceutical Research and Manufacturers of America (PhRMA), organized interest groups can and do dramatically change the ratio between the costs and benefits of participation in the political markets for policies.

A number of interest groups have become extraordinarily influential demanders of health policies. Necessary to successful participation in the political marketplace for any interest group is that its costs (including the costs of organizing the group, representing members' interests to policymakers, and providing sufficient resources of money and time to policymakers to exert real influence on them) be lower than the value of the benefits the group is able to obtain for its members through its impact on the menu of policies that affect the members.

From iron triangles to policy networks. Any policy domain, whether it is health or another domain such as defense, education, or welfare, attracts a set of participants, each of whom has some stake in the policies affecting the domain. Some of the participants, who are also known as stakeholders in a domain, demand policies; others supply policies. These stakeholders form a *policy community*, whose members share an interest in a common policy domain.

Traditionally, the membership of policy communities has included the legislative committees with jurisdiction in a policy domain, the executive branch agencies responsible for implementing policies in the domain, and the private interest groups in the domain. The first two categories are suppliers of the policies demanded by the third category. This triad of organized interests has been called an *iron triangle* because of its stability and ability to withstand attempts to make undesired changes in the status quo, at least when all three sides of the triangle are in accord on the appropriate policies in the domain.

The health policy domain, during the first half of the twentieth century, was dominated by a policy community that could be appropriately characterized as an iron triangle, one with a small number of powerful and concordant private sector members. Furthermore, the private sector members of the policy community, notably the AMA and the AHA, joined later by the American College of Physicians (ACP) and the American College of Surgeons (ACS), generally held a consistent view as to what the appropriate policies should be in this domain. These private sector members of the health policy community found sympathetic partners in the legislative committees and the implementing agencies for the most part. Together, they formed a formidable iron triangle. Their shared view of optimal health policy was that government should protect the interests of health care providers and not intervene in the financing or delivery of health care (Starr 1982; Wilsford 1991; Peterson 1993). Under these rather straightforward conditions, it was relatively simple for the suppliers and demanders of policies to satisfy each other.

The latter half of the twentieth century, however, has been a different story. The original members of the policy community are still in place, but fundamental differences have emerged in their views of optimal health policy. Medicine no longer speaks through the single voice of the AMA; organizations such as the ACP and the American Academy of Family Physicians (AAFP) can and sometimes do support different policy choices. The AHA now is joined in policy debates by the diverse preferences of organizations representing the specific interests of teaching hospitals, public hospitals, for-profit hospitals, or some other subset of hospitals.

Not only do the traditional members of the health policy community find themselves split over questions of optimal health policy, the community has been considerably enlarged as new interest groups have formed and joined (Salisbury 1990). Business is the major new member. It, too, is split, in this case primarily along large and small employer lines. Other newer members of the health policy community represent consumer interests. But the interests of consumers are not uniform, nor are the policy preferences of their interest groups.

There is no longer a block of homogeneous interests driving health policy decisions. Instead, the health policy community today "is heterogeneous and loosely structured, creating a network whose broad boundaries are defined by the shared attentiveness of participants to the same issues in the policy domain" (Peterson 1993, 409). There is an important difference between shared attentiveness to issues and agreed upon positions on the issues.

The members of the policy network in the health domain today compete with each other, often fiercely, regarding the design of the nation's optimal health policy. Some stakeholders derive benefits from the status quo or are threatened by changes in the status quo; other stakeholders want to change things because the status quo either harms them or offers them few, if any, benefits. This policy network of heterogenous interests is highly fluid and unstable (Smith 1994). These characteristics of today's health policy community make it very difficult for the suppliers of health policies to discern what the demanders really want, or which of their diverse demands they should attempt to meet.

The suppliers of health policies

Since policies are made in the executive, legislative, and judicial branches of government, the list of potential suppliers of health policies—the policymakers—is lengthy. Members of each branch of government play roles as suppliers of policies in the political market, although the roles are played in very different ways.

Legislators as suppliers. Few aspects of the political marketplace are as interesting, or as widely observed and studied, as the question of what motivates elected politicians. This intense interest is imbedded in the desires of the demanders of policies to exert influence over these suppliers of policies as they pursue desired policies. While neither extreme fully reflects the motivations of many, if any, real politicians, the end points on a continuum of behaviors potentially exhibited by politicians can be represented by those who seek to maximize the *public interest* and by those who seek to maximize their *self-interest* (Marmor and Christianson 1982).

A politician at the public-interest extreme would always seek policies that maximize the public interest, although the real public interest might not always be easy to identify. A politician whose motivations lie at the self-interest extreme would always behave in a manner that maximizes self-interest, whether that be reelection, money, prestige, power, or whatever appeals to the self-serving person.

In the political marketplace, legislators can be found all along the continuum between extreme public- and self-interest motivations. Some observers are quick to ascribe self-interest motives to all legislators. Feldstein (1988), for example, speaking of legislators, asserts that "their actions are undertaken to benefit themselves; only as a byproduct may they also benefit the public" (18). The actions of most legislators, most of the time, are more likely to reflect a complex mixture of the two motivations, with exclusively self-interest or public-interest motives dominating decisions only rarely.

Motives aside, legislators are key suppliers of policies, especially of policies in the form of statutes or laws. In this market, legislators play central roles in supplying policies demanded by their various constituencies. Rational legislators constantly make calculations about the benefits and costs, and to whom, of their policymaking decisions, and, factoring in the interests they choose to serve, make their decisions accordingly. Their calculations are made much more complicated when the costs and benefits of a particular decision affects many different people in different ways.

In effect, most policies create winners and losers, with the gains enjoyed by some people coming at the expense of others. While it may be something of an overgeneralization, it is fair to say that most of the time, most legislators in such situations will seek to maximize their own net political gains because reelection is an abiding factor in their decisions and behaviors. That is, they may find that the best thing for them is to permit the winners their victory, but not by a huge margin so as to cushion the impact on the losers. For example, consideration of a policy to increase health care services for an underserved population at the expense of other people could result in any number of outcomes: few services at relatively low cost; more services at higher costs; many services at very high costs. Facing such a decision, policymakers often opt for the provision of a meaningful level of services, but one far below what could have been provided and at a cost below what would have been required for a higher level of services.

Executives and bureaucrats as suppliers. Members of the executive branch also play important roles as suppliers of policies. Presidents, governors, and other high-level executives propose policies in the form of proposed legislation and push legislators to enact their preferred policies. Top executives, as well as executives and managers in charge of departments and agencies of government, make policies in the form of rules and regulations used to implement statutes and programs. In this, they are direct suppliers of policies. Elected and appointed executives and managers are joined in the rulemaking role by career bureaucrats who also participate in this process and thus become suppliers of policies in the political marketplace. The motivations of these participants in the supplying of policies differ.

Elected and politically appointed officials of the executive branch often are affected by the same self-interest/public-interest dichotomy that affects legislators; reelection concerns often directly influence the decisions of these people as well. They are also calculative regarding the net political gains available through their positions and actions regarding various policies. As a result, the motivations and behaviors of elected and politically appointed officials are often quite similar to those of legislators in the workings of the political marketplace.

However, there are some important differences between the motivations and behaviors of elected and appointed members of the executive branch of a government and the elected members of its legislature. The most fundamental of these differences, in regard to domestic as opposed to foreign policies, derives from the fact that the executive branch generally bears greater responsibility for the state of the economy than does the legislative branch. Presidents and governors and their top appointees are held accountable for the condition of the economy in the nation or in the various states more explicitly than the Congress or state legislatures. This is not to say that legislators escape this responsibility altogether. However, most people, if they do not lay the blame at the feet of the executive branch entirely, are more likely to hold the Congress or the state legislature collectively responsible than they are to blame their individual legislators.

The concentration of responsibility for the condition of the economy in the executive branch heavily influences the decision making that takes place there. Because of the close connection between government's budget and the state of the economy, the budget implications (i.e., deficit increasing or deficit reducing implications) of every policy decision will be carefully weighed in the executive branch. Not infrequently, positions on health policies will differ between the legislative and executive branches because members in the two branches attach different degrees of importance to the budget implications of the decisions they face.

As noted earlier, career bureaucrats in the executive branch also participate in rulemaking, making them direct suppliers of policies. They also collect, analyze, and transmit information about policy options and initiate policy proposals in their areas of expertise. In these ways, they are important participants in the policymaking role of the executive branch. Their motivations and behaviors differ both from those of legislators and from elected and appointed members of the executive branch.

The behaviors and motivations of career bureaucrats are often quite analogous to those of employees in the private sector. Workers in both the public and private sectors seek to satisfy certain of their personal needs and desires through their work. This can obviously be categorized as serving their self-interest in both cases. But government employees are no more likely to be totally motivated by self-interests than are private sector workers. Most workers in both sectors are motivated by the same mixture of self-interest and public interest (usually called community interest when the reference is to workers in the private sector) that influence elected and appointed government officials.

Having said this, it is also fair to point out that most career bureaucrats watch a constantly changing mix of elected and senior government officials—with an equally dynamic set of policy preferences—parade past them, while they remain as the most permanent human feature of government. It should surprise no one that career bureaucrats develop strong senses of identification with their home departments or agencies or that they develop attitudes of protectiveness toward these homes. This protectiveness is most visible in the relationships between government agencies or departments and those with legislative oversight, including authorization, appropriation, and performance review responsibilities toward them. Many career bureaucrats equate the well being of their agencies, in terms of their size, budgets, and prestige, with the public interest. This is obviously not necessarily the case.

The judiciary as supplier. The judicial branch of government also is a supplier of policies. Whenever a court interprets an ambiguous statute, establishes judicial procedure, or interprets the U.S. Constitution, it makes policies. These activities are not conceptually different from legislators enacting statutes or members of the executive branch establishing rules and regulations for the implementation of the statutes. All three activities fit the definition of policies in that they are authoritative decisions made within government for the purpose of influencing or directing the actions, behaviors, and decisions of others.

The heart of the judiciary's ability to supply policies lies in its role in interpreting the law. This power includes the power to declare federal and state laws unconstitutional—that is, to declare laws enacted by the legislative and executive branches to be null and void. The judiciary can also interpret the meaning of statutes, an important role since many statutes contain vague language, and they can decide how statutory laws are to be applied to specific situations. And particularly important to their role as suppliers of policies, the courts can exercise the powers of nullification, interpretation, and application to the rules and regulations established by the executive branch and within the government's regulatory agencies themselves.

One notable example of the role of the courts in American health policy is found in the treatment of the health insurance industry under the nation's antitrust laws. In 1944, the U.S. Supreme Court ruled that insurance was interstate commerce and thus subject to federal antitrust laws. But the insurance industry convinced the Congress that it faced financial ruin if subjected to antitrust laws. For example, to accurately determine rates, the industry argued that it needed to be able to pool data on claims and losses. Congress passed the McCarran-Ferguson Act (P.L. 79-15) in 1945, which included what was intended to be a temporary three-year exemption for the health insurance industry from federal antitrust laws. Since then, however, courts have interpreted a rather ambiguous section of the law in such a way that the exemption has been perpetuated and regulation of the health insurance industry has remained almost exclusively a responsibility of the states.

Recently, this matter has received renewed attention. As reported in *The New York Times* of 22 June 1993 (Pear 1993b), the House Judiciary Committee concluded that "lax oversight of the insurance industry, coupled with no possibility of antitrust enforcement, has led to the proliferation of anticompetitive practices" (A1). In the same account, state officials who testified before the Judiciary Committee were reported to have told the committee that the 1945 law "had bred a culture of collusion, leaving insurers free to fix rates, carve up markets, restrict coverage and insist that consumers buy products like prescription drugs from selected suppliers" (Pear 1993b, A9).

The courts are involved in numerous and diverse areas of health policy: termination of treatment, environmental responsibilities, approval of new drugs, mental health law, genetics, antitrust, and on and on. It is generally acknowledged that because the pursuit of health in the

United States is so heavily influenced by laws and regulations that the courts are a major factor in the development and implementation of health policies (Christoffel 1991). The courts include not only the federal court system, but the systems of the 50 states and the territories. Each of these systems has developed in idiosyncratic ways. Each court system has a constitution to guide it, specific legislation to contend with, and its own history of judicial decisions.

Although the federal and state courts play significant roles as suppliers of policies, their behaviors and motivations, as well as their roles, differ significantly from the legislative and executive branches. In their wisdom, the drafters of the U.S. Constitution created the three branches and ensured under Article III the judicial branch's independence, at least largely so, from the other branches.

An independent judiciary facilitates adherence to the rules of the game by which all participants in the policymaking process must play. Federal judges are appointed rather than elected, and the appointments are for life. Consequently federal judges, once they occupy these roles, are not subject to the same self-interest concerns related to reelection that many other policymakers must face. This enhances their ability to act in the public interest, although the courts also "enforce the 'deals' made by effective interest groups with earlier legislatures" (Landes and Posner 1975, 894).

Within the context of the political marketplace, many participants seek to further their objectives, whether these be self-interest perhaps involving some economic advantage or public-interest involving certain participants' perception of what is best for the nation. In both cases, the outcome depends greatly on the relative abilities of participants in the exchanges within the marketplace to influence actions, behaviors, and decisions of other participants.

Power and influence in political markets

Influence in political markets, just as in private economic markets is "simply the process by which people successfully persuade others to follow their advice, suggestion, or order" (Keys and Case 1990, 38). But, to have influence one must also have power. Power, in the context of market relationships and exchanges, whether it occurs in economic or political markets, is the potential to exert influence. More power means more potential to influence others. Therefore, to understand influence, one must first understand power.

Those who wish to exert influence in the political marketplace must first acquire power, utilizing the various sources of such power as might be available to them. The classic scheme for categorizing the several bases of interpersonal power includes legitimate, reward, coercive, expert, and referent power (French and Raven 1959).

Legitimate power derives from a person's position in a social structure or in an organization; this form of power is also called formal power or authority. It exists because societies find it advantageous to assign certain powers to individuals in order for them to be able to perform their jobs effectively. Thus, elected officials, appointed executives, and judges, as well as health professionals, corporation executives, and union leaders, and many other participants in the political marketplace possess certain legitimate power that accompanies their social or organizational positions.

Reward power is based on the person's ability to reward compliance with the behaviors that are sought in others. Reward power stems in part from the legitimate power a person holds; superiors in organizations have reward power over their subordinates. But reward power comes in many forms. Within organizations it includes the obvious: pay increases, promotions, work and vacation schedules, recognition of accomplishments, and such status symbols or perks as club memberships and office size and location. In economic markets, reward power lies in the hands of consumers by virtue of their buying power. In political markets, reward power is more likely to come in the form of such political capital as favors that can be provided or exchanged, specific influence with particular individuals or groups, and whatever influence can be stored for later use. *Coercive power* is the opposite of reward power and is based on a person's ability to withold or to prevent someone from obtaining desired rewards.

Expert power derives from possessing expertise valued within the political marketplace, such as expertise in solving problems or performing crucial tasks. Expert power is personal to the individual who possesses the expertise, which distinguishes it from legitimate, reward, or coercive power that is delegated to people by the organizations in which they work or by the social structure within which they operate. However, individuals may be granted these forms of power because they possess considerable expert power. People with expert power often occupy formal positions of authority in the areas of their expertise, but they may also simply be trusted advisors or associates of other participants in the political marketplace.

Referent power derives from the fact that some people engender admiration, loyalty, and emulation from others to such an extent that they gain power to influence these other people as a result. In the marketplace for policies, this form of power is sometimes called *charismatic power*. Charismatic power usually belongs to a select few *elected* and highly visible people. These people typically have very strong convictions about the correctness of the vision they have for the nation or state they represent, great self-confidence in their ability to realize the vision, and are perceived by their followers as legitimate agents of change. It is very rare for a person to be able to gain sufficient power to heavily influence followers simply from referent or charismatic power, even in political markets where charisma is highly valued.

Importantly, for the use and impact of power, these five bases of power in the political marketplace are interdependent. They can and do complement or conflict with each other. People who are in a position to use reward power, and who do so wisely, can strengthen their referent power. Conversely, people who abuse coercive power will quickly weaken or lose their referent power and very likely increase not only the number of but the intensity of feelings among their enemies. Effective participants in the marketplace for policies—those who succeed at translating their power into influence—tend to be fully aware of the sources of their power and to act accordingly. Effective participants seem to be those who "understand—at least intuitively—the costs, risks, and benefits of using each kind of power and are able to recognize which to draw on in different situations and with different people" (Morlock, Nathanson, and Alexander 1988, 268).

What distinguishes the ability of some people to effectively use the power to which they have access (that is, to translate power into influence in the political marketplace) are their interpersonal and political skills. It is not enough to have access to power; one must also know how to use it to influence others. Mintzberg (1983), perhaps as much as anyone, has recognized this important fact. He attributes success in using power largely to a person's relative political skills, which he defines as

> the ability to use the bases of power effectively—to convince those to whom one has access, to use one's resources, information, and technical skills to their fullest in bargaining, to exercise formal power with a sensitivity to the feelings of others, to know where to concentrate one's energies, to sense what is possible, to organize the necessary alliances. (Mintzberg 1983, 26)

Having examined the concept of political markets for policies, and having identified the demanders and suppliers who interact in these markets, we can now consider the intricate process through which policies are made. As will be seen, the motivations and behaviors of the participants in this process follow closely those outlined above. This makes the process more understandable and predictable, although in the playing out of the process there are always a few surprises.

The Public Policymaking Process

Figure 2.1, which is a simplified schematic model of the public policy-making process in the United States, illustrates the process as distinctly cyclical. The circular flow of the relationships among the various components of the model is one of its most important features. Policymaking is an on-going process in which almost all decisions are subject to subsequent modification. Another important feature shown in the model is that the entire process is influenced by factors that are external to the process. This makes the policymaking process an open system—one in which the process interacts with its external environment. This is shown by the impact of biological, cultural, demographic, ecological, economic, ethical, psychological, social, and technological inputs on the policy-making process. Legal and political inputs are assumed to occur within the context of the process itself. A third important feature of the model is that the various component parts of the policymaking process are highly interactive and interdependent. These important features are examined in more depth in subsequent chapters.

One feature that the model does not show, but one that is important to recognize if the policymaking process is to be understood, is the political nature of the process in operation. While there is a belief among many people—and a naive hope among still others—that policymaking is a predominantly rational decision-making process, this is not the case. The process would be simpler and better if it were driven exclusively by fully informed consideration of the best ways for policy to support the nation's pursuit of health, by open and honest debate about such policies, and by the rational selection of policies based strictly on their ability to contribute positively to the pursuit of health. But the process is not driven exclusively by these considerations.

In reality, a wide range of other intervening considerations invade and influence the policymaking process. Interest group preferences and influence, political bargaining and vote trading, and ideological biases are among the most important of these other factors. Truth and rationality do indeed play parts in health policymaking. On a good day, they will gain a place among the flurry of political considerations. But, as Brown (1991) has noted, "It must be a very good and rare day indeed when policy makers take their cues mainly from scientific knowledge about the state of the world they hope to change or protect" (20). While the model depicted in Figure 2.1 does not show these political considerations, they will receive attention in our discussion of the model and its component parts throughout the remainder of the book. This should be kept in mind as we consider the operation of the policymaking process.

The process includes three interconnected phases: *policy formulation*, which incorporates activities associated with agenda setting and subsequently with the development of legislation; *policy implementation*, which incorporates activities associated with rulemaking and policy operation; and *policy modification*. The formulation phase (making the decisions that lead to legislation) and the implementation phase (taking actions and making additional decisions necessary to implement legislation) are bridged by the formal enactment of legislation, which shifts the cycle from its formulation to implementation phases.[1]

Policies, once enacted as laws, must be implemented. Responsibility for this rests mostly with the executive branch, which includes many departments (e.g., the U.S. Departments of Health and Human Services and Justice). It also includes the activities of a number of independent federal agencies such as the Consumer Product Safety Commission and the Federal Trade Commission. These entities in the executive branch of government exist to implement the policies embodied in legislation. But it is important to remember that some of the decisions made *within* these organizations as they implement policies become policies themselves.

For example, rules and regulations promulgated in order to implement a law are policies just as are the laws whose implementation the rules support. Similarly, judicial decisions regarding the applicability of laws to specific situations or regarding the appropriateness of the actions of implementing organizations are decisions that are included in the nation's health policy according to the definition given in Chapter 1. Importantly, policies are established within both the policy formulation and policy implementation phases of the process.

The policy modification phase exists because perfection cannot be achieved in the other phases and because policies are established and exist in a dynamic world. Suitable policies made today may become inadequate with future biological, cultural, demographic, ecological, economic, ethical, psychological, social, and technological changes.

Policy modification, which is shown as a feedback loop in Figure 2.1, might entail nothing more than minor adjustments made in the implementation phase or modest amendments to existing legislation. In some circumstances, however, the outcomes and consequences of implementing certain policies can feed back all the way to the agenda-setting stage of the process. For example, the challenge of formulating policies to contain health care costs facing policymakers today is in part an outgrowth of the success of previous policies that expanded access and subsidized an increased supply of human resources and advanced technologies to be used in the provision of health services.

It should be kept in mind as the separate components of the policymaking model are examined individually and in greater detail in subsequent chapters that the model depicts a political process, a process that is cyclical in its operation, a process that is heavily influenced by factors external to the process, and a process whose component parts are highly interactive and interdependent.

Ethics in the policymaking process

Because the health policymaking process is controlled by people, it is influenced by various mixes of altruism and egoism. Human control of the process also means that its outcomes and consequences are affected by the ethics of those who participate in the process. Ethics plays an important part in the making of policy, but only a part. As has been noted by Beauchamp and Childress (1989):

> The making of policy is more complex than applying principles and rules. No ethical theory composed of abstract principles and rules can dictate policy, because it cannot contain enough specific information or guidance. The application of moral principles must take account of problems of efficiency, cultural pluralism, political procedures, uncertainty about risk, noncompliance by patients, and the like. The principles provide the moral background for policy, but the policy itself must be informed by empirical data and by special information available in the fields of medicine, biology, law, psychology, and so on. (13–14)

Ethics plays a part in the policymaking process in two equally important ways. Ethical principles can guide the original development of new policies. But ethics can also be used to legitimately criticize policies already made and thus can form the basis for their amendment or modification (Thompson 1985). Ethical behavior, for any and all participants in policymaking, is guided by four philosophical principles: respect for the autonomy of other people, justice, beneficence, and nonmaleficence.

The concept of autonomy is based on the notion that individuals have the right to their own beliefs and values and to the decisions and choices that further these beliefs and values. The ethical principle of *respect for autonomy* undergirds much of the formal system of government the founders of our nation envisioned. Beauchamp and Childress (1989) have pointed out that there is no fundamental inconsistency or incompatibility between the autonomy of individuals and the authority of government so long as government's authority does not exceed the limits set by those who are governed. In this context, autonomy pertains to the rights of citizenship in the United States. Specifically, autonomy pertains to the rights of individuals to independent self-determination regarding how they live their lives and to their rights regarding the integrity of their bodies and minds. Respect for autonomy in health policymaking will influence issues such as liberty rights, privacy, and individual choice, including behavioral or lifestyle choices.

Policymaking that reflects the principle of respect for autonomy can sometimes be better understood in contrast to its opposite—paternalism. Paternalism implies that someone else knows what is best for other people. Polices guided by a preference for autonomy limit paternalism. One of the most vivid examples of the kind of policies that result from adherence to the principle of autonomy in health policymaking is the 1990 Patient Self-Determination Act (P.L. 101-508). This policy is designed to give individuals the right to make decisions concerning their medical care, including the right to accept or refuse treatment, and the right to formulate advance directives regarding their care. These directives are a means by which competent individuals give instructions about their health care that are to be implemented at some later date should they then lack the capacity to make medical decisions. In concept, this policy gave people the right to exercise their autonomy in advance of a time when they might no longer be able to actively exercise the right.

The principle of respect for autonomy includes several other elements that are especially important in guiding ethical behavior in policymaking. One of these is telling the truth. Respect for people as autonomous beings implies honesty in relationships with them. Closely related to honesty in such relationships is the element of confidentiality. Confidences broken in the policymaking process can impair the process. A third element of the autonomy principle that is important to the policymaking process is fidelity. This means doing one's duty and keeping one's word. Fidelity is often equated with keeping promises. When participants in the policymaking process tell the truth, honor confidences, and keep promises, the process is more ethically sound than if these things are not done.

A second ethical principle of significant importance to policymaking is *justice*. The concept of justice, which is derived from political philosophy, impacts directly on the policymaking process and on policies themselves. In Rawls' (1971) words, "One may think of a public conception of justice as constituting the fundamental charter of a well-ordered human association" (5). Much of its impact on policies and on policymaking hinges on defining justice as fairness (Rawls 1971). The principle of justice also includes the concept of desert: justice is done when a person receives that which he or she deserves (Beauchamp and Childress 1989). The practical implications for health policymaking of the principle of justice are felt mostly in terms of distributive justice— that is, in terms of fairness in the distribution of health care benefits and burdens in society. The key policy question, deriving from attention to the ethical principle of justice, is, of course, "What is fair?"

The various participants in the health policymaking process hold varying opinions on the issue of what is a fair or just distribution of the benefits and burdens involved in the pursuit of health in American society. Useful insight into the range of possible views on fairness in this matter can be gained from considering the three most prominent general theories of justice.

Egalitarian theories of justice hold that all should have equal access to both the benefits and burdens arising from our pursuit of health and that fairness requires a recognition of different levels of need. The influence of the egalitarian view of justice can be seen in a number of health policies. Policies intended to remove discrimination in the provision of health care services reflect the preference for equality. Policies intended to provide more resources to those thought to need them most (e.g., Medicare for the elderly or Medicaid for the poor) are also based on an egalitarian view of fairness. Libertarian theories hold that fairness requires a maximum of social and economic liberty for individuals. Policies that favor unfettered markets as the means of distributing the benefits and burdens reflect the libertarian theory of justice. Utilitarian theories hold that justice is best served when public utility is maximized. This is sometimes expressed as the greatest good for the greatest number. Many public health policies, including those pertaining to restricting pollution, ensuring safe workplaces, and controlling the spread of communicable diseases, have been heavily influenced by a utilitarian view of what is just in the distribution of the benefits and burdens arising from the American pursuit of health.

The principle of justice provides much of the underpinning for all health policies, whether they are in the allocative or regulatory categories. Allocative policies that adhere closely to the principle of justice (called distributive justice in this context) allocate resources according to the provisions of a morally defensible system rather than through arbitratry or capricious decisions. Regulatory policies guided by the principle of justice impact fairly and equitably on those to whom the regulations are targeted. A mark of distinction in the policymaking process in the United States is that a dynamic legal system exists to help ensure that the principle of justice is respected in the formulation and implementation of policies and to serve as an appeals mechanism for those who believe the process has not adequately honored this principle.

Two other ethical principles have direct relevance to policymaking—beneficence and nonmaleficence. *Beneficence* in policymaking means acting with charity and kindness. This principle is incorporated into acts through which benefits are provided; thus beneficence characterizes most allocative policies. But beneficence also includes the more complex concept of balancing benefits and harms, for using the relative costs and benefits of alternative decisions and actions as one basis on which to choose from among alternatives. The growing emphasis on cost effectiveness in medical care and the development of policies to support this will increasingly call into play the principle of beneficence in developing ethically sound policies. Policymakers who are guided by the principle of beneficence make decisions that maximize the net benefits to society as a whole.

Nonmaleficence, a principle with deep roots in medical ethics, is exemplified in the dictim *primum non nocere*—first, do no harm. Policymakers who are guided by the principle of nonmaleficence make decisions that minimize harm to society as a whole. The principles of beneficence and nonmaleficence are clearly reflected in health policies that seek to ensure the quality of health care services and products. Such policies as those establishing peer review organizations (PROs) to review the quality of care given to Medicare patients and the policies that the Food and Drug Administration use to ensure the safety of pharmaceuticals are examples.

Conclusion

Health policies, like those in other domains, are made through a highly complex, interactive, and cyclical process that incorporates formulation, implementation, and modification phases of activities. The process is played out in the context of the political marketplace, where demanders and suppliers of policies interact. The participants in the health policymaking process are diverse; they include elected and appointed members of all three branches of government as well as the civil servants who staff the government, groups of individuals and organizations to whom policies are targeted, organized interest groups, the media, researchers and consultants, and, of course, the public. The interests of these participants are rarely coincident, often they are in conflict, and always the activities of any participants affect and are affected by the activities of other participants. Thus, policymaking is very much a human process, a fact with great significance for the outcomes and consequences of the process.

There are competing theories about how public policymaking occurs in the United States. At the opposite ends of a continuum sit public interest and self-interest theories. Policies made strictly in the public interest would be those that result when all participants act according to what they believe to be the public interest. Policies made strictly through a process driven by the self-interest of the participants would reflect an intricate calculus of the interplay of various self-interests. Policies resulting from these two hypothetical extremes of the way people can behave in the policymaking process would likely be very different. In truth, the constitutional system of government in the United States establishes a process within which competing interests can struggle to establish their particular definition of the public interest, at least temporarily until a new set of competing interests redefine the public interest. In a nation of diverse interests, there can be no such thing as *the* public interest.

In reality, various health policies reflect different mixes of public-interest and self-interest influences. On balance, however, it appears that self-interest has exerted more influence than public interest in policy-making related to our pursuit of health. Perhaps the best evidence for this view is the coexistence of the extremes of excess (e.g., high incomes of physicians and managers, overinsurance, esoteric technologies, and duplicate facilities) and deprivation (e.g., lack of insurance and inadequate access to basic health services) that have resulted from the nation's health policy to date. Public policymaking in the health domain in the United States is a remarkably complex and interesting process, but clearly it has also been an imperfect process. The intricacies of the process are explored more thoroughly in the following chapters, where each of its interconnected phases is examined in more detail.

Note

1. The conceptualization of the public policymaking process as a set of interrelated phases has been used by a number of authors, although there is considerable variation in what the phases of activities are called in these models as well as in their comprehensiveness. For a good generic example, see G. D. Brewer and P. de Leon, *The Foundations of Policy Making*, Homewood, IL: Dorsey, 1983. P. A. Paul-Shaheen has used such a model to analyze health policymaking specifically; see "Overlooked Connections: Policy Development and Implementation in State-Local Relations," *Journal of Health Policy, Politics and Law* 15, no. 4 (Winter 1990): 833–56.

References

Beauchamp, T. L., and J. F. Childress. *Principles of Biomedical Ethics*, 3d ed. New York: Oxford University Press, 1989.

Brown, L. D. "Knowledge and Power: Health Services Research as a Political Resource." In *Health Services Research: Key to Health Policy*, edited by E. Ginzberg, 20–45. Cambridge, MA: Harvard University Press, 1991.

Christoffel, T. "The Role of Law in Health Policy." In *Health Politics and Policy*, 2d ed., edited by T. J. Litman and L. S. Robins, 135–47. Albany, NY: Delmar Publishers Inc., 1991.

Feldstein, P. J. *The Politics of Health Legislation: An Economic Perspective*. Ann Arbor, MI: Health Administration Press, 1988.

French, J. R. P., and B. H. Raven. "The Basis of Social Power." In *Studies of Social Power*, edited by D. Cartwright, 150–67. Ann Arbor, MI: Institute for Social Research, 1959.

Greenberger, D., S. Strasser, R. J. Lewicki, and T. S. Bateman. "Perception, Motivation, and Negotiation." In *Health Care Management: A Text in Organization Theory and Behavior*, 2d ed., edited by S. M. Shortell and A. D. Kaluzny, 81–141. New York: John Wiley & Sons, 1988.

Keys, B., and T. Case. "How to Become an Influential Manager." *The Executive* 4, no. 4 (November 1990): 38–51.

Landes, W. M., and R. A. Posner. "The Independent Judiciary in an Interest-Group Perspective." *The Journal of Law and Economics* 18, no. 3 (December 1975): 875–901.

Longest, B. B., Jr. "Inter-Organizational Linkages in the Health Sector." *Health Care Management Review* 15, no. 1 (Winter 1990): 17–28.

Marmor, T. R., and J. B. Christianson. *Health Care Policy: A Political Economy Approach*. Beverly Hills, CA: Sage Publications, 1982.

Mintzberg, H. *Power In and Around Organizations*. Englewood Cliffs, NJ: Prentice-Hall, 1983.

Morlock, L. L., C. A. Nathanson, and J. A. Alexander. "Authority, Power, and Influence." In *Health Care Management: A Text in Organization Theory and Behavior*, 2d ed., edited by S. M. Shortell and A. D. Kaluzny, 265–300. New York: John Wiley & Sons, 1988.

Pear, R. "Clinton's Health-Care Plan: It's Still Big, But It's Farther Away." *The New York Times*, 13 June 1993a.

———. "Insurers Facing Closer Scrutiny in Clinton Plan." *The New York Times*, 22 June 1993b.

Peterson, M. A. "Political Influence in the 1990s: From Iron Triangles to Policy Networks." *Journal of Health Politics, Policy and Law* 18, no. 2 (Summer 1993): 395–438.

Rawls, J. *A Theory of Justice*. Cambridge, MA: The Belknap Press of Harvard University Press, 1971.

Salisbury, R. H. "The Paradox of Interest Groups in Washington—More Groups, Less Clout." In *The New American Political System*, edited by A. King. Washington, DC: The American Enterprise Institute, 1990.

Smith, M. J. *Pressure, Power and Policy: Policy Networks and State Autonomy in Britain and the United States*. Pittsburgh, PA: University of Pittburgh Press, 1994.

Starr, P. *The Social Transformation of American Medicine*. New York: Basic Books, 1982.

Thompson, D. "Philosophy and Policy." *Philosophy and Public Affairs* 14, no. 2 (Spring 1985): 205–18.

Wilsford, D. *Doctors and the State: The Politics of Health in France and the United States*. Durham, NC: Duke University Press, 1991.

Figure 3.1 A Model of the Public Policymaking Process in the United States: The Policy Formulation Phase

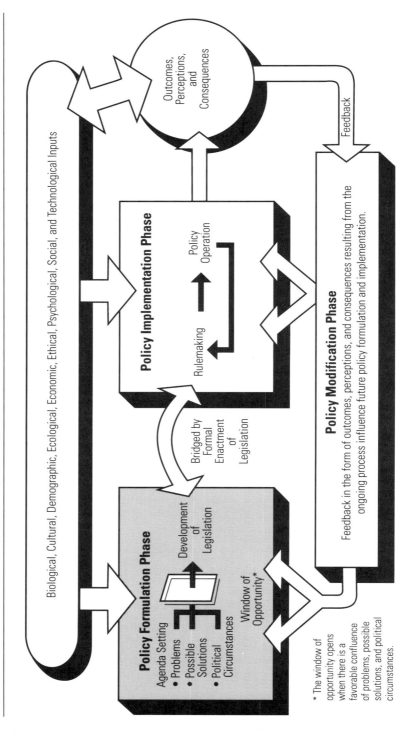

3

Policy Formulation

The formulation phase of health policymaking includes two distinct and sequentially related sets of activities—agenda setting and legislation development. These activities of policy formulation, depicted in the highlighted portion of Figure 3.1, are the focus of this chapter.

The myriad decisions that comprise the nation's health policy eventually emerge from a diverse array of problems, possible solutions to the problems, and dynamic political circumstances. At any point, there are many problems or issues related to health. Many of them have possible solutions; often they have alternative solutions, each of which can have supporters and detractors. The existence of problems and potential solutions is overlaid by diverse political interests. The ways in which particular issues emerge from this mix to advance to the next stage in the policymaking process is an important feature of the process and is termed *agenda setting*.

Once health policy issues rise to prominent places on the political agenda, they can, but do not always, proceed to the next stage of the policy formulation phase, *development of legislation*. At this stage, specific legislative proposals go through a process involving a carefully prescribed set of steps that can, but do not always, lead to policies in the form of new laws or statutes or, as is more often the case, amendments to previously enacted statutes. Only a small fraction of the potential universe of policy issues emerge from the agenda-setting activity surrounded by the circumstances necessary to provide the impetus for them to advance to the point of having specific legislation developed to address the issues. And, even then, only some of the attempts to enact legislation are successful. The path for legislation can be long and arduous.

Agenda Setting

Kingdon (1984) was the first to describe agenda setting in public policymaking as a function of the confluence of three "streams" of activities:

problems, possible solutions to the problems, and political circumstances. In his conceptualization, when all three flow together in a favorable alignment, a "window of opportunity" (see Figure 3.1) is created through which a policy issue emerges from the pack and activity shifts to the development of legislation to address the issue. Current policies such as those pertaining to environmental protection, licensure of health professionals and institutions, and funding for AIDS research exist because these issues had previously emerged as sufficiently important that policies to address them were developed.

But the mere existence of problems in these areas was not sufficient to ensure the development of legislation intended to address them. The existence of problems, even serious ones such as high costs and uneven access to needed health services, does not invariably lead to policies that solve them. There must also be potential solutions to the problems and the political will to enact specific legislation pertaining to the problems. Obviously, agenda setting is crucial to the nature of the nation's health policy and to every specific policy within the larger set. Agenda setting is best understood in the context of its three key variables—problems, possible solutions, and political circumstances.

Problems

The breadth of this initiating variable in agenda setting can be seen in the range of possible public sector decisions (policies) that can affect the pursuit of health. Remember, as was discussed in Chapter 1, that health is determined by several factors acting in combination: the physical, sociocultural, and economic environments in which people live; their lifestyles, behaviors, and genetics; and the type, quality, and timing of health care services that they receive. Beyond this, as shown overarching Figure 3.1, the biological, cultural, demographic, ecological, economic, ethical, psychological, social, and technological aspects of American life feed into the agenda-setting activity. These inputs join with the outcomes, perceptions, and consequences of the ongoing policymaking cycle (notice the feedback loop from the outcomes component to the agenda-setting component of Figure 3.1) to continuously supply those responsible for setting the nation's policy agenda with a massive pool of contenders for a place on that agenda.

Problems that require policy solutions may find their place on the agenda along any of several paths. Some problems emerge because the trends in certain variables eventually reach unacceptable levels. Growth in such variables as the number of people with AIDS, the number who are uninsured, and costs in the Medicare program are examples of trends that eventually reached levels at which policymakers had to address the underlying issues. Other problems emerge by virtue of some specific event that forces attention. Examples include medical waste products washing up on beaches or the discovery of a new drug for treating AIDS that is so expensive few people can purchase it on their own. Problems can also be spotlighted by their widespread applicability to many people (e.g., the high cost of prescription medications affects millions of Americans) or by their sharply focused impact on a small but powerful group whose members are directly affected (e.g., the high cost of medical education).

Some problems gain their place on the agenda or have their hold on a place strengthened because they are closely linked to other problems that already occupy secure places on the policy agenda. President Clinton's efforts to firmly establish a linkage between inflation in the health sector and the nation's growing budget deficit problem as part of his push to have health reform legislation developed in 1993–1994 is an example of this phenomenon. In this instance, the linkage of one policy issue (health care cost inflation) to another (deficit reduction) strengthened the political prospects for the development of legislation intended to contain health care costs.

On occasion, problems emerge along several of these paths more or less simultaneously. Such problems occupy places of considerable prominence on the agenda of items that might spur the development of legislation. The present concern over health costs, for example, has emerged along a number of mutually reinforcing paths. In part, the cost problem is prominent in the health policy community because trend data regarding health costs is now startling. Recall Table 1.3 in Chapter 1, which showed that on the present trajectory, 18.1 percent of the gross domestic product (GDP) will be devoted to health care by the year 2000, up from 14.4 percent in 1993. Related predictions include that about 30 percent of federal outlays (excluding interest), up from about 18 percent in 1993, will be for health costs by then (U.S. Congressional Budget Office 1992). Data on such trends reinforce a widespread acknowledgement of the problem and focus the attention of some of those who pay for health care, especially government and the business community. Finally, the cost problem has been linked to another significant item on the nation's policy agenda, the mushrooming federal deficit.

The combination of these circumstances regarding the health cost problem reinforce each other and help explain why this issue now occupies such a prominent place in the minds of policymakers. It is generally the case that issues that eventually do lead to the development of legislation are those broadly identified as important and urgent; otherwise, they languish at the bottom of the agenda or never are placed on the agenda at all. The cost of health care is so firmly planted in the policy agenda at this time that we can be certain that it will continue to spur the development of additional policies intended to solve the problem (Jencks and Schieber 1992; Fuchs 1993; Helms 1993).

Possible solutions

The second variable in agenda setting is the existence of possible solutions to problems. The mere existence of problems, no matter how serious or widely acknowledged they are, is not sufficient to trigger the active development of legislation to address them. For this to happen, there must also exist possible solutions to the problems. This variable involves generating ideas for solving problems, refining the ideas, and ultimately, selecting from among the options.

In the late 1980s and early 1990s, the search for solutions to the problem of health care costs led to the active—indeed, feverish—consideration of a number of possible solutions to the problem. A very rich and diverse menu of possible solutions for policymakers' review evolved. Ordered roughly along a dimension of less to more radical departure from the status quo, the possible policy approaches to solving the health care cost problem that were developed or proposed fit generally into four categories.

- *Policy incrementalism*, including such ideas as waiving state mandates in health insurance coverage, reducing administrative costs by standardizing insurance claim forms, instituting reforms to slow the costs of large malpractice awards and the defensive medical practices used to avoid them, and prohibiting physicians from referring patients to facilities that the physicians own, comprised one category.

- *Managed competition*, under which vertically integrated networks of providers would compete on the basis of price and quality for large pools of insured people, represented another category. While there were variations in the managed competition models, the basic components usually had government establishing a standard benefit package and quality standards and imposing community rating on the establishment of prices.[1]

- *Global budgets*, proposed by some to be established at the national level and by others at the level of states, featured placing caps on total expenditures on health care at some predetermined level represented yet a third distinct category of possible solutions for the health care cost problem.[2]

- *Single-payer systems*, such as exist in Canada or Great Britain, were the preferred solution to the cost problem by some people. Such systems feature government's assumption of the role of single payer for all health services and its use of the resultant market power to hold down costs.

The masssive scope of the health care cost problem and the variety of economic interests involved in any effort to solve the problem drove the development of an unusually large and diverse set of alternative solutions to this problem. Reflecting the intense interest in solving the problem of health care costs, more than 100 legislative proposals seeking to address some aspect of the health cost problem were introduced in the 102d Congress during 1991 and 1992. This was followed by the introduction of still other proposals in 1993, including the Clinton administration's plan, The Health Security Act, to make health coverage universal in the United States and to control the growth in health care costs.

While the menu of alternative solutions to problems is not usually as large or diverse as the one that developed regarding the need to control health care costs, there are almost always alternative possible solutions to the problems that face policymakers. Without at least one solution, issues do not advance in the policymaking process. When there are many alternatives, each with its opponents and proponents, advancement can be slowed as the relative merits of the competing alternatives are considered.

Decision making regarding alternative solutions

The existence of problems and possible, or alternative, solutions to them are two prerequisites for use of the classical, rational model of decision making that is outlined in Figure 3.2. This model of decision making reflects the basic pattern of the decision-making process typically utilized in both the private and public sectors in the United States. However, differences frequently arise in the process when the criteria to be used in evaluating alternative solutions to problems are introduced.

Some of the criteria used as the bases for evaluating and comparing alternative solutions to problems in both the private and public sectors are of course the same or very similar. Typically, the criteria set in both sectors includes consideration of whether a particular solution will actually solve the problem; whether it can be implemented within available resources and technologies; its costs and benefits relative to other possible solutions; and the results of an advantage-to-disadvantage analysis of the alternatives. But the most substantive difference between the criteria sets used in making decisions in the two sectors lies in the application of political concerns and considerations.

Public policies require that decisions reflect political sensitivity to the public at large and to special interest groups to a far greater extent than most decisions made in the private sector. This helps explain the

Figure 3.2   The Rational Model of Decision Making

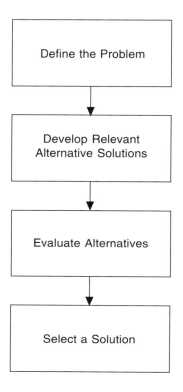

considerable importance of the third variable in agenda-setting, political circumstances.

Political circumstances

This third variable in creating a window of opportunity through which issues move to the point at which legislation is developed includes such factors as the public attitudes, concerns, and opinions surrounding an issue; the preferences and relative ability to influence political decisions of various groups that have an interest in the issue; the positions of key political leaders in the executive and legislative branches of government on the issue; and the other competing items on the policy agenda. The last item is often overlooked, but it is an important political variable. When the nation is involved in serious threats to its national security or its civil order, for example, or when a state is in the midst of a sustained recession, health policy will be treated differently than when policy-makers are less preoccupied with other, perhaps more urgent, concerns.

Creating a political thrust forceful enough to have policymakers attempt to do something substantive about a policy issue is often the most problematical variable in having an issue emerge from the pack of competing issues. This elusive element often keeps the window of opportunity closed, preventing movement to the active development of legislation to address the issue. This circumstance is not particularly surprising, in part because the form of government in the United States lends itself to political stalemate. Out of fear of government, the nation's founders created a government more suited to inaction than to action (Morone 1990).

Another important factor in explaining why political circumstances so often prevent progression to policy development is the nature of the American electorate. While voters usually do not have the opportunity to vote directly on policies, they do have the opportunity to vote on policymakers. Thus, policymakers are interested in what the voters want, even when it is not easy to discern what they want. And, often, it is very difficult to judge the electorate's position on issues. One of the great myths of a democratic society is that its voters, when confronted with tough choices, will ponder the choices carefully and express their preferences to their elected officials, who can then factor these opinions into their decisions. Sometimes this happens, but even when it does, the American electorate is not homogeneous. Opinions on any health policy issue are usually mixed.

Polls of potential voters can help sort out conflicting opinions, but polls are not always straightforward undertakings. Complicating the use of polls is the fact that on many issues the individual voter's opinion is subject to evolutionary change. Yankelovich (1992) points out that the public's thinking on difficult problems that might be addressed through public policies evolves through predictable stages, beginning with awareness of the problem and ending with judgments about its solution. In between, they explore, with varying degrees of success, the problem and alternative solutions. Where voters are along this continuum of stages has a great deal to do with their views on both problems and their solution.

Interest group involvement in setting the health policy agenda

One of the most significant features of the political economy of the United States, in regard to health policy, is the fact that while individuals tend to be keenly interested in their own health and that of others they care about, the public's interest in specific health policies tends to be rather diffuse. As was pointed out in Chapter 2, this stands in contrast to the interests of those who earn their livelihoods in this domain or who stand to gain specific and advantageous benefits from the health domain. Their interests are not at all diffused. They are, in fact, highly concentrated. This phenomenon is not unique to health. Indeed, it is generally the case that the interests of those who earn their livelihoods in any industry or economic sector are more concentrated than the interests of those who merely use its outputs; and they are far more concentrated than those who have only incidental or occasional interaction with the domain.

One result of the existence of concentrated interests is the formation of organized interest groups. These groups seek to influence the formulation, implementation, and modification of policies for the purpose of providing the group's members some advantage. While the membership of the U.S. Congress numbers 535 people, there are now more than 1,200 organized interest groups actively seeking to influence their health policy decisions.

Since all interest groups seek policies that favor their members, their agendas and behaviors are rather predictable. Feldstein (1988) argues, for example, that all health care provider interest groups seek through legislation to increase the demand for members' services, limit competitors, permit members to charge the highest possible prices for their services, and lower their members' costs of operating as much as possible. Likewise, an interest group representing a group of health care consumers would seek policies that minimize the costs of the services to the members, ease their access to the services, increase the availability of the services, and so on.

Interest groups play powerful roles in setting the nation's health policy agenda, as they do subsequently in the development of legislation and in the implementation and modification of policies. These groups can play their roles proactively by seeking to stimulate new policies that serve the interests of their members. They can, alternatively, play their roles reactively by seeking to block changes or advances in public policies that they do not believe serve their members' best interests. Interest groups are an inherent part of the public policymaking process in the United States. And they are especially ubiquitous in the health sector.

Individual physicians can join and have some of their interests represented by the American Medical Association (AMA). Nurses can join the American Nurses' Association (ANA). Hospitals can join the American Hospital Association (AHA), which seeks to serve its member organizations' needs and preferences. Teaching hospitals can join the Council of Teaching Hospitals (COTH), children's hospitals can join the National Association of Children's Hospitals and Related Institutions, and investor-owned hospitals can join the Federation of American Health Systems

(FAHS). The other groups of professional and institutional providers are also represented by interest groups.

In addition, a number of nonprovider groups with concentrated interests have formed special interest groups. Examples include the Association of American Medical Colleges (AAMC), the Blue Cross and Blue Shield Association, the Health Insurance Association of America (HIAA), the Pharmaceutical Research and Manufacturers of America (PhRMA), and the Industrial Biotechnology Association (IBA). Even subsets of the population can join a group that seeks to serve their interests. For example, the American Association of Retired Persons (AARP) is a powerful association to which many of the nation's older citizens belong. Other consumer-oriented interest groups include Citizen Action, the National Council of Senior Citizens, Families U.S.A., and the Consortium for Citizens With Disabilities.

The influential role of chief executives in agenda setting

Another, and very important, element in the political circumstances variable in agenda setting is the role of the chief executive—the president, governor, or mayor. In cases where these individuals enjoy popularity, they can easily play preeminent roles in agenda setting. Kingdon (1984) attributes the influential role of presidents (his point also applies to other chief executives) in agenda setting to certain institutional resources inherent in the executive office. These politically advantageous resources include the ability to present a unified administration position on issues, which stands in stark contrast to the legislative branch where opinions and views tend to be heterogeneous, and the executive's ability to command public attention. Properly managed, this latter ability can foster substantial public pressure on legislators in support of the executive's preferences and viewpoints.

Lammers (1991) highlights the ability of chief executives to perform "issue raising activities" as crucial to their ability to influence agenda setting. He notes that the development of legislation is "generally preceded by a variety of actions which first create a widespread sense that something needs to be done, and—as action becomes imminent—that something will be done" (Lammers 1991, 96). Issues can be raised in a number of ways including in speeches and addresses. This can be especially potent in such highly visible contexts as State of the Union or State of the State addresses.

Candidates for the presidency are sometimes quite specific in their campaigns on various health policy issues, sometimes even to the point of endorsing specific legislative proposals (Fishel 1985). Examples include the emphasis given to enactment of the Medicare program by

Presidents Kennedy and Johnson in their campaigns and President Clinton's highly visible commitment to fundamental health care reform as a central theme of his 1992 campaign.

Another issue-raising mechanism favored by some executives is the appointment of special commissions or task forces. President Clinton used this tactic in the 1993 appointment of the President's Task Force on Health Care Reform. He greatly enhanced the visibility, and the effectiveness, of the task force by naming his wife, Hillary Rodham Clinton, to chair the group.

It should be noted here that chief executives are usually in positions to be very influential in each phase of the policymaking process. We have concentrated thus far on their role in agenda setting, but they are also well positioned to help focus the Congress on the development of legislation and to motivate members to continue their legislative work on favored issues even when the legislators face enormous competing demands on their time and attention. In addition, chief executives, as will be discussed in Chapter 4, are central to the implementation of policies by virtue of their positions atop the executive (or implementing) branch of government. They also play crucial roles in modifying policies, as will be discussed in Chapter 5.

The role of research and analysis in health policy agenda setting

The American health policy agenda is determined by the confluence of problems, potential solutions to the problems, and political circumstances variables. Research, especially some that is conducted in the increasingly important interdisciplinary field of health services research, contributes heavily to both problem identification and the development of possible solutions. As has been noted by Shortell and Reinhardt (1992):

> Health services research can play an important role in the process of policy formulation and implementation. After all, that process inevitably proceeds on the basis of deeply held perceptions that may have been shaped by personal experience, by anecdotes, or by formally structured information from a variety of sources. Sometimes these perceptions may be an accurate reflection of the facts. At other times, however, they will rest on the most casual of empirical bases and border on folklore. Finally, at yet other times these perceptions may be deliberately manipulated through biased information supplied by particular interest groups. Health services research, when properly conducted, attempts to free itself from the imperatives of any one particular interest group. Instead, at its best it seeks to bring the perceptions of decision makers as closely as possible to the facts of a situation. (3–4)

The kinds of issues and questions to which research can help supply valuable information for the purpose of helping to formulate health
policies are driven by the determinants of health that were identified in
Chapter 1: the environmental conditions under which people live, their
behaviors and genetics, and the health care system that serves them.
Within each of these areas, many questions and issues are currently receiving attention from the research community.

In the area of the health care system, for example, the diversity of
important questions is illustrated by the following categorization of a set
of research questions that will remain important to health policy formulation throughout the 1990s:

- *Access to health services:* How can an appropriate and affordable
  set of health services be made available to all citizens?

- *Organization of health services:* How can health services be organized most effectively and efficiently?

- *Financing health services:* How can the funds necessary to operate
  a health system be collected most effectively and efficiently?

- *Reimbursement of health services:* How can health services providers be paid for their services most effectively and efficiently?

- *Cost of health services:* How can the cost of health services be controlled more effectively and efficiently?

- *Quality of health services:* How can the quality of health services
  be assessed and ensured most effectively and efficiently?

- *Special populations:* How can the health care needs of special
  population groups be met most effectively and efficiently?

- *Ethical and legal issues:* What are the ethical and legal issues that
  need to be addressed in providing access to affordable health
  services of an appropriate quality in the most effective and efficient manner possible? (Crane, Hersh, and Shortell 1992, 370–71)

There are three distinct ways in which research can influence health
policymaking: documentation, analysis, and prescription (Brown 1991).
All three mechanisms can exert influence in the agenda-setting stage of
the larger policymaking process depicted in Figure 3.1.

As we have said, agenda setting begins with the existence of problems. Moynihan (1970) once observed that "society cannot act on social
problems until it knows it has them, and it often does not know it has
them until it can *count* them" (30). Thus, the first role of research in
policymaking is *documentation*—that is, the gathering, cataloging, and
correlating of facts that depict the state of the world that policymakers
face (Brown 1991). For example, only after the documentation of the dangers of tobacco smoke, which in the early days was almost totally based

on the correlation between smoking and cancer, were policymakers pushed into action on this health issue. As another example, present efforts to modify policies or to develop new policies to help address the needs of those who lack health insurance follow considerable documentation of the existence and magnitude of this problem.

A second way in which research informs, and thus influences, policymaking is through *analysis* of what does and does not work. Often taking the form of demonstration projects intended to provide a basis in fact for determining the feasibility, efficacy, or just plain workability of a possible policy intervention, analysis can reveal much of value to policymakers.

Finally, in Brown's (1991) typology, the third way in which research influences policymaking is through *prescription*. Policies, even if they are formulated mainly on political grounds, must also stand the test of plausibility. Research, which helps attest that a particular course of action being contemplated by policymakers might not boomerang or embarrass them, can therefore make a significant contribution to policymaking.

One thing that research cannot do is to clearly delineate *the best* solutions to problems—at least, it cannot do this very often. In part this is because the complexity of many health issues outstrips the power of available research tools and designs. But this is also due partly to the tendency of researchers to focus on narrow rather than broad conceptualizations of problems. This narrow, and often very limiting focus, is taken because it enhances the probability that one's work will be funded and/or published. But it also means that the work might not contribute very much to solving complex policy challenges. One consequence of a large volume of research that explores bits and pieces of issues is that often a policymaker with a particular perspective on an issue can find one or more researchers whose work is consistent with the perspective. This lends itself to a situation in which research stimulates, or at least facilitates, the making of more—not fewer and better focused—policies.

Health policy agenda setting and the poly-policies phenomenon

The poly-policies phenomenon represents a common condition in public policymaking and derives from the fact that, in a pluralistic society where difficult problems exist and where clear-cut solutions are rare, there are likely to be a number of different "sides" to any particular issue or problem, each with its supporters and detractors. The number, ratio, and intensity of these supporters and detractors is determined by the impact of the problem and its solution on those who take positions. One consequence of this phenomenon is a severe crowding of the health policy agenda.

As policymakers seek to serve the needs and preferences of different interests, or "sides," on particular issues or problems, the eventual result can be a set—at times, a large and diverse set—of policies. This is the poly-policies phenomenon. And the set, even though focused on a particular issue or area, can be almost devoid of internal consistency. American health policy offers many examples of situations in which sets of policies, developed over time and through the involvement of many policymakers seeking to serve different interests, result in patterns of policies that, while related, are riddled with incompatibilities and inconsistencies. This is the poly-policies phenomenon at work.

The nation's mix of policies regarding the production and consumption of tobacco products, a mix that simultaneously encourages and discourages tobacco use, provides a good example of policies at cross-purposes. A closely related situation arises when the poly-policies phenomenon results in a set of policies with a consistent purpose but with different emphases about which people can disagree. The nation's mix of AIDS policies, for example, reflect this phenomenon.

On the issue of combatting AIDS, some policies have been developed to support the clinical study of the human immunodeficiency virus (HIV) and its impact on humans. Other policies simultaneously support the search for an effective vaccine. Still others support education about the transmission of the virus and attempt to change human behaviors that help spread the virus. There is significant disagreement within the health policy community about the appropriate mix of these types of policies and the share of available funds that should be allocated to each. This discord exists in spite of the fact that all of these policies share the ultimate purpose of minimizing the suffering and death caused by HIV.

The poly-policies phenomenon, which is similar to what Foote (1991) has termed "polyintervention," can also be observed in the pattern of American policies related to medical technology. Policymakers have sought to serve the goal of spreading the benefits of new medical technology and, concurrently, to serve such goals as protecting the public from unsafe technologies and attempting to slow the growth in overall health care costs through controlling the explosive growth of new technologies. The result is a large group of technology-related policies that seek both to foster and to inhibit the development, diffusion, and use of medical technology in the United States. Table 3.1 is a poly-policies matrix of current key policies that affect medical technology.

There are several reasons for the ambivalence about whether policy should foster or inhibit technology that is reflected in the pattern of policies shown in Table 3.1. All of the reasons have to do with the particular perspective on the issue that one or more interest groups hold.

Table 3.1   The Current Matrix of Key Policies Affecting Medical Technology

| Stage | Examples of Policies that | |
	Foster	Inhibit
Development	NIH, DOD, NASA, NSF, and other science and biomedical funding	FDA regulation
	Tax credits for private R&D	Product liability statutes
Diffusion	Patent and intellectual property laws	Certificate-of-need programs
	Cost- or charge-based insurance	Capitation-based insurance (such as HMOs)
	Antitrust laws	Technology assessment and outcomes research
Use	Medicare and Medicaid	Prospective payment system for Medicare program and state-imposed limits on Medicaid programs
	Tax breaks for employer-provided health insurance	Limitations on insurance coverage for experimental technology
	VA health care funding	

Note: Assessments with a similar theme can be found in Foote (1991) and Kessler, Pape, and Sundwall (1987).

Some of the ambivalence no doubt results from the fact that it is not definitively clear what role technology actually plays in the rising cost of health care. After all, these costs result from an intricately woven web of actors, actions, and inactions, including: increased longevity of the population; inadequate attention to prevention; labor-intensiveness in health care delivery, coupled with high earnings of professional, administrative, and technical health care workers; as well as the use of sophisticated and costly technology and extensive insurance coverage (U.S. Department of Commerce 1993).

While many analysts suspect that, among these and other variables, technology is a major culprit in rising costs (Nyman 1991), and most agree that it plays a part, its exact impact is not well established (Neumann and Weinstein 1991). Nevertheless, analysts generally agree that at least part of the increase in these costs can be "ascribed to the growth of new and expensive medical technology" (U.S. Congressional Budget Office 1992, 21). In particular, technology is linked with insurance as an especially potent interactive force for rising costs:

> Newly developed technologies have driven up both costs of care and the demand for insurance, while also expanding the range of services for which consumers demand insurance. At the same time, expanding insurance coverage, which includes more people as well as a growing array of health care inputs, has provided an increased incentive to the R&D sector to develop new technologies, and a growing incentive for subsets of consumers who could benefit from particular new technologies to seek a wider definition of what would be covered by insurance. (Weisbrod 1991, 546)

Coincident with the uncertainties about the precise role of technologies in rising health costs, there is little doubt about the fact that although technology may be costly, it also produces health benefits for people. These benefits of medical technology, often available in combinations, include:

- Diagnosis and treatment for previously untreatable diseases (e.g., immunosuppressive drugs that make organ transplants possible, and AZT for people with AIDS)
- Improved diagnoses and treatments (e.g., an array of imaging technologies, clot-dissolving tPA for myocardial infarction, the genetically engineered drug EPO, which accelerates the body's production of red blood cells)
- Increased patient comfort and safety (e.g., lithotripsy in place of surgery or, better yet, drugs that dissolve stones without surgery or lithotripsy).

The combination of concerns about the cost impact of medical technologies and desires to ensure that their benefits are available no doubt play a significant part in the pattern of fostering and inhibiting policies shown in Table 3.1. To these concerns and desires can be added a third possible reason for the coexistence of fostering and inhibiting policies—medical technology's economic role.

Although medical technology generates costs for consumers, for whom it may also produce health benefits, it also clearly generates enormous economic benefits. These benefits are in the form of revenues for producers and for those who use the technology in their work and in the form of taxes on these revenues that are paid to government. Indeed, technological advances, including medical technology, have long been seen as vital to the nation's economic growth and place on the world's economic stage by business people and public officials alike (Dutton 1988). Medical technology plays an important role not only in the nation's domestic economy, but since this technology is competitive worldwide, it is an increasingly important element in its trade balance position.

Given the diversity of interests that stand to be served by supporting or inhibiting medical technology, and the abiding commitment of policymakers to link their positions on particular issues to the positions of influential constituencies, it is not surprising that a poly-policies pattern such as the one depicted in Table 3.1 emerges. In fact, it is rarely possible to isolate single policies about health issues because the complexity of the problems and of the political circumstances surrounding the problems do not lend themselves to such neatness. Instead, health policies tend to exist in a rather seamless mosaic of numerous related, and sometimes contradictory, policies.

However, each individual policy, at least those in the form of laws or statutes, is created through a legislative process that generally grinds along addressing a number of policy issues at any given time. In situations where the existence of a problem is widely acknowledged, where possible solutions have been identified and refined, and where favorable political circumstances exist, a window of opportunity opens, albeit sometimes only briefly. Through this window, an issue moves forward and the development of legislation intended to address the issue is initiated (see Figure 3.1). When this happens, policymakers use a dynamic, highly interactive process through which they seek to convert ideas and hypotheses into concrete policies.

The Development of Legislation

This section contains a simplified and abbreviated outline of the very complex process through which legislation is developed at the federal level. With modifications, which vary from state to state, the legislative process in the states is similar, at least in a general sense, to the federal process outlined here. The process consists of a carefully ordered set of steps. The tangible final products of the legislative process are *laws* or *statutes*. At the federal level, these are first printed in pamphlet form called *slip law*. Later, laws are published in the *Statutes at Large* and eventually incorporated into the *United States Code*. The series of steps outlined below apply whether legislation is completely new or whether, as is so often the case, it represents the amendment of prior legislation.

Drafting and introducing legislative proposals

The legislative process begins with legislative proposals, called *bills*. (Proposed legislation can also be introduced as a *resolution*. As a practical matter, there is little difference between a bill and a resolution and they will not be differentiated here.) The pathway from the drafting of bills to enacted statutes is long and arduous. Only a small fraction of the bills introduced in a Congress are actually passed. Those not passed die at the end of the Congress (the two annual sessions spanning the term of office of members of the House of Representatives) in which they were introduced and must be reintroduced in the next Congress if they are to be considered further.

　　Legislative proposals can be drafted by any senator or representative, and these legislators' staffs are usually instrumental in drafting legislation. When issues are especially complex, the Legislative Counsel's Office in the Senate or House of Representatives can be called on for assistance in drafting bills. Proposed legislation can also be drafted by others, including people in the executive branch, private groups such as associations or other health interest groups, or even individual citizens. No matter who drafts legislation, however, only members of the Congress can officially sponsor proposed legislation, and the legislative sponsors are ultimately responsible for the language in the bills they sponsor. Commonly, a bill will have multiple sponsors—up to 25 in the House of Representatives and an unlimited number in the Senate.

Introduction and referral of proposed legislation

Proposed legislation, in the form of a bill, is introduced by members of the Senate or House of Representatives who have chosen to sponsor or cosponsor the bill. On occasion, identical bills are introduced in both the Senate and the House for simultaneous consideration. When bills are introduced in either chamber of the Congress, they are assigned a sequential number (e.g., HR-1 or S-1), based on the order of introduction, by the presiding officer and are referred to the appropriate standing committee for further study and consideration. The assignment to the appropriate committee depends on the content of the bill and the jurisdiction of the committees and of their subcommittees. Sometimes the content makes the assignment to more than one committee appropriate; in these cases the bill can be assigned to more than one committee either jointly or, more commonly, sequentially. The Clinton administration's Health Security Act was introduced simultaneously in the House and Senate on 20 November 1993 as HR-3600 and SB-1757. Because of its magnitude, the bill was referred, jointly, to ten House Committees and two Senate Committees for consideration and debate.

Legislative committees and subcommittees

Both the Senate and House of Representatives are organized into committees and subcommittees. Ideally, this facilitates the division of work and the orderly consideration of proposed legislation. In reality, however, the committee structure itself can sometimes present or exacerbate problems. As Tribe (1973), in an unusually harsh assessment of the committee system, observed, "The existing system of specialized committees, riddled with rivalries and fragmented jurisdictional division, cannot be relied upon to provide the focus without which public concern is just so much undirected energy" (609). And as Blank (1988) has noted, "The present committee system fails to address matters that cut across its divisions" (160). Even in the face of these shortcomings, however, the committee structure is a fundamental feature of the development of legislation.

The majority party in each chamber controls the appointment of committee and subcommittee chairpersons. It also appoints the majority of each committee or subcommittee's members and assigns most of the staff for each committee. The chairpersons of committees and subcommittees exert great power in the legislative process because they determine the order in which and the pace at which legislative proposals are considered by their respective committees or subcommittees. The professional staff serving committees and subcommittees, by virtue of expert knowledge, are key participants in the legislative process. A number of committees and subcommittees are involved in health affairs. The most important in terms of health policy are:

- Senate Finance Committee, which has jurisdiction over all bills related to the Social Security Act, including Maternal and Child Health, and Medicare and Medicaid; and which includes the Subcommittee on Health for Families and the Uninsured, and the Subcommittee on Medicare and Long-Term Care.

- Senate Labor and Human Resources Committee, which has jurisdiction over all bills related to the Public Health Service Act, the Federal Food, Drug and Cosmetic Act, and the Developmental Disabilities Assistance and Bill of Rights Act; also authorizes the National Science Foundation; while this committee has subcommittees, all health legislation is considered by the full committee.

- Senate Appropriations Committee, which includes the Subcommittee on Labor, Health and Human Services, Education, and Related Agencies, which has jurisdiction over appropriations for the Department of Health and Human Services except for the Food and Drug Administration, the Indian Health Service, and the Office of Consumer Affairs; and the Subcommittee on Veterans Affairs, Housing and Urban Development, and Independent Agencies, which has jurisdiction over appropriations for the Department of Veterans Affairs.

- Senate Committee on Veterans Affairs, which has jurisdiction over all legislation related to programs in the Department of Veterans Affairs; this committee does not have subcommittees.
- House Ways and Means Committee, which includes the Subcommittee on Health, which has jurisdiction over most bills related to the Social Security Act, including Medicare Part A.
- House Energy and Commerce Committee, which includes the Subcommittee on Health and the Environment, which has jurisdiction over all bills related to the Public Health Service Act and selected programs in the Social Security Act, including Maternal and Child Health, Medicare Part B, and Medicaid.
- House Appropriations Committee, which includes the Subcommittee on Labor, Health and Human Services, Education, and Related Agencies, which has jurisdiction over appropriations for the Department of Health and Human Services except for the Food and Drug Administration, the Indian Health Service, and the Office of Consumer Affairs; and the Subcommittee on Veterans Affairs, Housing and Urban Development, and Independent Agencies, which has jurisdiction over appropriations for the Department of Veterans Affairs.
- House Veterans Affairs Committee, which includes the Subcommittee on Hospitals and Health Care, which has jurisdiction over legislation involving veterans' hospitals, medical care, treatment of veterans, and VA research.

Depending on whether the chairperson of a committee has assigned a bill to a subcommittee or not, either the full committee or the subcommittee can hold hearings. Members of the executive branch, representatives of interest groups, and other individuals are permitted to present their views and recommendations on the legislation under consideration at these hearings.

After such hearings, committee or subcommittee members will *mark up* the bill. This term comes from the procedure of going through the bill line by line and making changes through a process of amending the original bill. Sometimes when similar bills or bills addressing the same issue have been introduced, they are combined in the marking-up process. In cases in which a subcommittee is involved, when the subcommittee completes the marking-up process, it *reports out* the bill to the full commit-tee with jurisdiction. When no subcommittee is involved, or after a full committee reviews the work of the subcommittee, the full committee reports out the bill, this time to the floor of the Senate or House for a vote.

House or senate floor action on proposed legislation

Following approval of a bill by the full committee with jurisdiction, the bill is discharged from the committee along with a *bill report* that contains a great deal of information about the bill's history and the committee's reasons for approving the bill. The House or Senate receives the bill from the relevant committee and places it on the legislative calendar for floor action. A bill can be further amended in debate on the floor of the House or the Senate. However, because such great reliance is placed on the com-mittee process in both chambers, amendments to bills proposed from the floor require considerable support.

Bills, once passed in either the House or Senate, are sent to the other chamber, where the process of being referred to a committee and per-haps then to a subcommittee is repeated and where there may be another process of hearings, mark-up, and eventual action. If the bill is again re-ported out of committee, it goes to the involved chamber's floor for a final vote. If passed in the second chamber, any differences in the House and Senate versions of a bill must be resolved before the bill is sent to the White House for action by the president. The Congress uses conference committees to iron out any differences in the versions of bills passed by the House and Senate.

Conference committee action on proposed legislation

The procedure for resolving differences in a bill that has been passed by both chambers of the Congress is the establishment of a conference com-mittee that is charged to resolve the differences (Van Beek 1994). Confer-ees usually are the ranking members of the committees that reported out the bill in each chamber. If they can reach agreement on resolving the differences, a conference report is written, and this is then voted on by both houses of the Congress. In the event that the conferees cannot reach agreement, or if either house does not accept the report, the bill dies. However, if both chambers accept the conference report the bill is sent to the president for action.

Presidential action on proposed legislation

The president has several options regarding proposed legislation that has been approved by both the House and Senate. The bill can be signed, in which case it immediately becomes law. The bill can be vetoed by the president, in which case it must be returned to Congress along with an explanation of the basis for rejection. By two-thirds vote in both houses of the Congress, a presidential veto can be overridden. The president's third option is to neither veto nor sign the bill. In this case, the bill becomes law in ten days, but the president has made a political statement of disapproval of the legislation. Finally, when proposed legislation is received by the president near the close of a Congress, the president can *pocket veto* the bill by doing nothing until the Congress is adjourned. In this case, the bill dies.

Conclusion

The policy formulation phase of policymaking involves agenda setting and the development of legislation. Agenda setting is a set of activities through which a suitable configuration of problems, possible solutions to the problems, and political circumstances permit certain policy issues to progress along to the point of legislation development.

The development of legislation follows a carefully prescribed choreography that includes the drafting and introduction of legislative proposals, their referral to appropriate committees and subcommittees, House and Senate floor action on proposed legislation, conference committee action when necessary, and presidential action on legislation enacted by the legislature.

The point at which proposed legislation is formally enacted into law is the point of transition in the policymaking process from policy formulation to policy implementation. As shown in Figure 3.1, the formal enactment of legislation serves to bridge the formulation and implementation phases of the policymaking process and triggers the implementation phase of the process. Issues of implementation are considered in the next chapter.

Notes

1. As described by Helms (1993, xiii–xiv), "Managed competition refers to a concept of reform deriving from the analytical works of Alain C. Enthoven of Stanford University and Paul M. Ellwood with InterStudy and the Jackson Hole Group. A specific proposal known as the Jackson Hole proposal was developed by a group of health policy analysts and health industry leaders meeting in the home of Paul Ellwood in Jackson Hole, Wyoming. The proposal envisions a market where large, full-service health delivery organizations compete with each other on the basis of price and quality. Limits on the present tax-free nature of employer-provided health insurance and other

regulations would give consumers strong economic incentives to choose among these competing plans. Comparisons among the plans would be simplified by requirements that each plan offer and quote prices for a defined set of benefits. Additional benefits could be purchased by the consumer with after-tax dollars. The process of certifying the competing plans and collecting and publicizing the information about each plan's performance and annual price bids would be carried out by health alliances (called health care purchasing cooperatives in the Jackson Hole proposal) at the state or substate level. A national board would define the basic benefit package, the standards for the operation of the health alliances and the competing health plans, and collect data on the cost-effectiveness of various coverages in the basic benefit package. Federal subsidies based on income would allow poorer consumers and employers to purchase health insurance from one of the competing health plans" (reprinted with permission from *Health Policy Reform: Competition and Controls*, edited by R. B. Helms © 1993 by AEI Press). More information on managed competition can be found in P. M. Ellwood, A. C. Enthoven, and L. Etheredge, "The Jackson Hole Initiatives for a Twenty-First Century American Health Care System," *Health Economics* 1 (1992): 149–68; and A. C. Enthoven, "The History and Principles of Managed Competition." *Health Affairs* 12 (Supplement 1993): 24–48.

2. Again in the words of Helms (1993, xiv) regarding global budgets as a potential solution to the cost problem, "The concept can mean different things to different people. The central concept, however, is a national, or top-down, system of expenditure controls designed to reduce aggregate health spending to a lower rate of increase. Following Stephen F. Jencks and George J. Schieber (1992), global budgets differ from expenditure targets because they contain some formal mechanism to ensure that expenditures do not exceed the target amount during a current accounting period. Some form of aggregate controls are used in several European countries and Canada. The prospect of adopting some form of global budgeting in the United States raises a host of issues about how the targets would be set, how they would be handed down to state and local areas, and how they would be measured and enforced" (reprinted with permission from *Health Policy Reform: Competition and Controls*, edited by R. B. Helms © 1993 by AEI Press, p. xiv). In addition to several of the chapters in Helms (1993) and to Jencks and Schieber (1992), additional information on the global budget strategy can be found in S. H. Altman and A. B. Cohen, "The Need for a National Global Budget," *Health Affairs* 12 (Supplement 1993): 194–203; P. Starr, *The Logic of Health-Care Reform*, Knoxville, TN: Grand Rounds Press, 1992; and P. Starr and W. A. Zelman, "Bridge to Compromise: Competition under a Budget," *Health Affairs* 12 (Supplement 1993): 7–23.

References

Blank, R. H. *Rationing Medicine*. New York: Columbia University Press, 1988.
Brown, L. D. "Knowledge and Power: Health Services Research as a Political Resource." In *Health Services Research: Key to Health Policy*, edited by E. Ginzberg, 20–45. Cambridge, MA: Harvard University Press, 1991.

Crane, S. C., A. S. Hersh, and S. M. Shortell. "Challenges for Health Services Research in the 1990s." In *Improving Health Policy and Management: Nine Critical Research Issues for the 1990s,* edited by S. M. Shortell and U. E. Reinhardt, 369–84. Ann Arbor, MI: Health Administration Press, 1992.

Dutton, D. B. *Worse Than the Disease: Pitfalls of Medical Progress.* New York: Cambridge University Press, 1988.

Feldstein, P. J. *The Politics of Health Legislation: An Economic Perspective.* Ann Arbor, MI: Health Administration Press, 1988.

Fishel, J. *Presidents and Promises.* Washington, DC: Congressional Quarterly Press, 1985.

Foote, S. B. "The Impact of Public Policy on Medical Device Innovation: A Case of Polyintervention." In *The Changing Economics of Medical Technology,* edited by A. C. Gelijns and E. A. Halm, 69–88. Washington, DC: National Academy Press, 1991.

Fuchs, V. R. *The Future of Health Policy.* Cambridge, MA: Harvard University Press, 1993.

Helms, R. B., editor. *American Health Policy: Critical Issues for Reform.* Washington, DC: The AEI Press, 1993.

Jencks, S. F., and G. J. Schieber. "Containing U.S. Health Care Costs: What Bullet to Bite?" *Health Care Financing Review* 13, 1991 annual supplement (March 1992): 1–12.

Kessler, D. A., S. M. Pape, and D. N. Sundwall. "The Federal Regulation of Medical Devices." *New England Journal of Medicine* 317, no. 6 (6 August 1987): 357–66.

Kingdon, J. W. *Agendas, Alternatives, and Public Policies.* Boston: Little, Brown, 1984.

Lammers, W. W. "Presidential Leadership and Health Policy." In *Health Politics and Policy,* 2d ed., edited by T. J. Litman and L. S. Robins, 95–115. Albany, NY: Delmar Publishers Inc., 1991.

Morone, J. A. *The Democratic Wish: Popular Participation and the Limits of American Government.* New York: Basic Books, 1990.

Moynihan, D. P. *Maximum Feasible Misunderstanding.* New York: Free Press, 1970.

Neumann, P. J., and M. C. Weinstein. "The Diffusion of New Technology: Costs and Benefits to Health Care." In *The Changing Economics of Medical Technology,* edited by A. C. Gelijns and E. A. Halm, 21–34. Washington, DC: National Academy Press, 1991.

Nyman, J. A. "Costs, Technology, and Insurance in the Health Care Sector." *Journal of Policy Analysis and Management* 10, no. 1 (Winter 1991): 106–11.

Shortell, S. M., and U. E. Reinhardt. "Creating and Executing Health Policy in the 1990s." In *Improving Health Policy and Management: Nine Critical Research Issues for the 1990s,* edited by S. M. Shortell and U. E. Reinhardt, 3–36. Ann Arbor, MI: Health Administration Press, 1992.

Tribe, L. H. *Channeling Technology Through Law.* Chicago: Bracton Press, 1973.

U.S. Congressional Budget Office. *Economic Implications of Rising Health Care Costs.* Washington, DC: U.S. Government Printing Office, 1992.

U.S. Department of Commerce. "U.S. Industrial Outlook 1993." Washington, DC: U.S. Government Printing, 1993.

Van Beek, S. D. *Post-Passage Politics: Bicameral Resolution in Congress.* Pittsburgh, PA: University of Pittsburgh Press, 1994.

Weisbrod, B. A. "The Health Care Quadrilemma: An Essay on Technological Change, Insurance, Quality of Care, and Cost Containment." *Journal of Economic Literature* 29, no. 2 (June 1991): 523–52.

Yankelovich, D. "How Public Opinion Really Works." *Fortune* (5 October 1992): 102–8.

Figure 4.1 A Model of the Public Policymaking Process in the United States: The Policy Implementation Phase

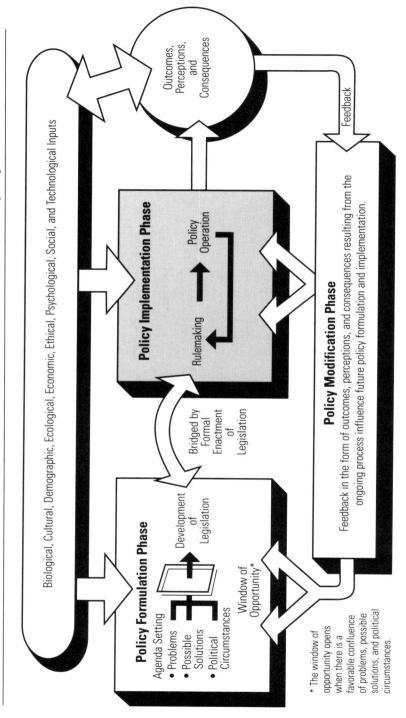

Biological, Cultural, Demographic, Ecological, Economic, Ethical, Psychological, Social, and Technological Inputs

Policy Formulation Phase

Agenda Setting
• Problems
• Possible Solutions
• Political Circumstances

Development of Legislation

Window of Opportunity*

Bridged by Formal Enactment of Legislation

Policy Implementation Phase

Rulemaking

Policy Operation

Outcomes, Perceptions, and Consequences

Policy Modification Phase

Feedback in the form of outcomes, perceptions, and consequences resulting from the ongoing process influence future policy formulation and implementation.

Feedback

* The window of opportunity opens when there is a favorable confluence of problems, possible solutions, and political circumstances.

4

Policy Implementation

In Chapter 2, the direct relationship between the policy formulation and policy implementation phases of policymaking was described. The formulation phase (making the decisions that lead to legislation) and the implementation phase (taking actions and making additional decisions necessary to implement legislation) are bridged by the formal enactment of legislation. Enactment shifts the focus from formulation to implementation.

The relationship between policy formulation and policy implementation is simple, direct—and very important. Policies, once enacted as laws, must be effectively implemented if they are to have any chance of exerting their intended impact on the human environment (including its physical, sociocultural, and economic components); human lifestyles, behaviors, and genetics; or on the health care system. This chapter specifically addresses the implementation of health policies (see the highlighted portion of Figure 4.1), although implementation cannot actually be quite so neatly separated from formulation.

In the implementation phase, much, but not all, of the responsibility in policymaking shifts from the legislative branch of government to the executive branch. Because implementation responsibility rests so heavily within the executive branch, many of executive branch departments, such as the U.S. Departments of Health and Human Services and Justice are involved, as are a number of independent federal agencies such as the Consumer Product Safety Commission and the Federal Trade Commission. These executive branch entities exist to implement the policies embodied in legislation.

Although the executive branch bears most of the responsibility for implementing policies, the legislative branch maintains an oversight responsibility and often a continuing appropriations responsibility in the implementation phase. There is also a judicial dimension to the implementation phase: administrative law judges hear the appeals of people or organizations that are dissatisfied with the way implementation of policies impacts on them. Legislation, as well as the rules made by those responsible for its implementation, can be challenged in the courts.

Very important to an understanding of policymaking, some of the decisions made *within* the executive branch organizations, as they implement policies, become policies themselves. For example, rules and regulations promulgated in order to implement a law are policies just as are the laws whose implementation the rules support. Similarly, decisions made in the judicial branch regarding the applicability of laws to specific situations or regarding the appropriateness of the actions of implementing organizations are decisions that are included in the nation's health policy according to our definition of policies as authoritative decisions made in the legislative, executive, or judicial branches of government that are intended to direct or influence the actions, behaviors, or decisions of others. By this definition, policies are established within both the policy formulation and policy implementation phases of the policymaking process.

As will be seen in this chapter, the implementation phase of the process involves managing human, financial, and other resources in such ways that the objectives and goals embodied in enacted legislation can be achieved by those responsible for implementation. The most important point in understanding policy implementation, as part of the larger cycle of policymaking, is that it should be viewed primarily as a *management* process. Management is a broad term that generally means "the process, composed of interrelated social and technical functions and activities, occurring in a formal organizational setting for the purpose of accomplishing predetermined objectives through the utilization of human and other resources" (Rakich, Longest, and Darr 1992, 6).

Depending on the scope of laws or programs, their implementation can be fairly simple and straightforward or can require massive managerial effort. President Lyndon B. Johnson observed that the preparations made for implementing the Medicare program (as contained in P.L. 89-97, which amended the Social Security Act in 1965) represented "the largest managerial effort the nation [had] undertaken since the Normandy invasion" (Iglehart 1992, 1,468).

The implementation phase of policymaking includes two separate but interrelated sets of activities—rulemaking and policy operation (see Figure 4.1). Both sets of activities are described in this chapter.

The Beginning of Implementation: Rulemaking

Enacted legislation seldom contains enough explicit language on how the legislation is to be implemented to completely guide the implementation process. Rather, laws are often vague on implementation details, leaving it to the implementing organizations to promulgate the rules needed to guide their operation. While the means through which the rules and regulations necessary for the implementation of laws are established varies among the levels of government, there are more similarities than differences. The federal process serves as a prototype and is the focus here.

The promulgation of rules, as a formal part of the implementation phase, is itself guided by certain rules. Key among these rules is the requirement that the organization responsible for implementing a law publish a Notice of Proposed Rulemaking (NPRM) in the *Federal Register*. A NPRM is, in effect, a draft of a rule or set of rules under development. Publication of this notice is an open invitation to all those in a relevant policy community—that is, those with an interest in the rules and regulations applicable to implementing a particular law—to react to proposed (draft) rules before they become final. Changes in proposed rules often result from this procedure. It is one of the most active points of involvement for interest groups and others who have a stake in a particular policy in the entire policymaking process.

Usually the link between legislation and the promulgation of necessary rules and regulations for its operation is fairly direct and the development of final rules takes place in a timely way. But this is not always the case. For example, Congress enacted the Hospital Survey and Construction Act (P.L. 79-725), also known as the Hill-Burton Act, after its sponsors, Senators Lister Hill and Harold Burton, in 1946. This law provided grants to build, expand, or modernize hospitals. It contained provisions that required grantees to provide "a reasonable volume of services to those unable to pay" and to make their facilities "available to all persons residing in their service areas." However, it was not until significant court action in the 1970s that the Department of Health, Education and Welfare (DHEW), now the Department of Health and Human Services (DHHS), promulgated effective rules governing these free care obligations. For 30 years, those responsible for implementing the law simply avoided issuing final rules that required hospitals to meet these obligations, apparently because they wished to avoid anticipated conflict with the hospital industry over the enforcement of these provisions of the law.

On occasion, especially when the development of rules and regulations is anticipated to be unusually difficult, or seems prone to spawn severe disagreements and conflicts, or when rules and regulations are anticipated to be subject to continuous revision, special provisions may be made regarding their development. For example, after passage of the Health Maintenance Organization Act (P.L. 93-222) in 1973, DHEW (now

DHHS) organized a series of task forces, including on them some members drawn from outside the implementing organization, to help develop the proposed rules for implementing the law. This strategy produced rules that were much more acceptable to those who would be affected by them than might have otherwise been the case.

Another strategy that is used to support rulemaking is the creation of advisory commissions to assist with the effort. For example, following enactment of the 1983 Amendments to the Social Security Act (P.L. 98-21), which established the prospective payment system (PPS) for reimbursing hospitals for the care of Medicare beneficiaries, Congress established the Prospective Payment Assessment Commission (ProPAC) to provide nonbinding advice to the Health Care Financing Administration (HCFA) in implementing the reimbursement system. Later, a second commission, the Physician Payment Review Commission (PPRC), was established to advise Congress and the HCFA regarding payment for physicians' services under the Medicare program. These commissions are quite useful in helping the HCFA to make required annual decisions regarding reimbursement rates, fees, and other variables in the operation of the Medicare program.

The link between legislators and implementors in rulemaking

The center of Figure 4.1 shows a bridge connecting the policy-formulation and policy-implementation phases of policymaking. This bridge is purposefully shown as a two-way connector between the two phases of the process. Implementing agencies are established and maintained and the people within them are employed to carry out the intent of legislation enacted by legislators. Legislators rely on the implementors to bring their legislation to life. The relationship is highly symbiotic.

Legislative oversight of implementing agencies, which is legitimized by congressional assignment of authorization, appropriation, and review responsibilities to certain legislative committees and subcommittees, provides a powerful linkage between legislators and implementors. Those with the authority monitor implementation and can identify situations in which legislative intent is not being realized in the implementation phase. (As will be discussed in Chapter 5, legislative oversight can also entail broader responsibilities including identification of situations in which modification of existing policies might be needed, or in which the results of one policy are in conflict with the desired results of other policies.) In the case of Congress, and with parallel arrangements in many of the states' legislatures, any committee with health jurisdiction can hold oversight hearings. However, the House Appropriations Committee and the Senate Appropriations Committee are especially prone to use the annual reviews of the budgets of implementing organizations and agencies to seek to influence implementation decisions.

Feldstein (1988) argues that the behaviors of implementors can best be understood by examining legislators' behaviors. In his view, "Both groups [legislators and implementors] attempt to maximize their political support. The groups that provide political support to the [implementing] agency are the same as those that provide political support to those legislators serving on the committee having jurisdiction over the agency. The only difference is that the agency also tries to provide the members of the legislative committee with political support" (Feldstein 1988, 26).

Both legislators and implementors seek political support of individuals and groups outside of government. As was seen in Chapter 2, the most influential of these potential supporters tend to be the well-organized interest groups. Thus, these interest groups seek to position themselves to exert influence over the formulation of policy *and* over its implementation.

The role of interest groups in rulemaking

Implementation of any complex health law or program provides many examples of what Thompson (1991) calls the "strategic interaction" that occurs between implementing organizations and affected interest groups during rulemaking. For example, among the numerous rules proposed in implementing the 1974 National Health Planning and Resources Development Act (P.L. 93-641) were some that sought to reduce obstetrical capacity in the nation's hospitals. One proposed rule, in 1977, called for hospitals to perform at least 500 deliveries annually or close their obstetrical units. Notice of this proposed rule elicited immediate objections, especially from hospitals in rural areas. The implementing organization (DHEW, now DHHS) received more than 55,000 written reactions to the proposed rule, almost all of them negative (Zwick 1978). As a result, the final rules were far less restrictive, in fact making no reference at all to a specific number of deliveries hospitals in rural areas should perform.

Because interest groups are so often the targets of rules established to implement health policies, they routinely seek to influence rulemaking. All policies have one or more target groups. Regulatory policies seek to prescribe and control the actions, behaviors, and decisions of targeted people and/or organizations. Allocative policies seek to provide income, goods, or services to targeted people and/or organizations at the expense of others. Target groups are the raison d'être of policies.

Target groups are very important in the implementation of policy. They tend not to be passive, and some are quite well organized and aggressive in seeking to influence both the formulation and implementation of policies that affect them. Many target groups are, in fact, interest groups. Associations representing hospitals, physicians, insurers, pharmaceutical manufacturers are examples of such groups. Obviously, target groups are quite diverse. Decisions that please some of them can easily displease others. All target groups have wants and preferences that they would like to have addressed through policy. This gives rise to the lobbying that permeates the political marketplace in which health policy is made in the United States. One consequence of the diversity among target groups is impetus for the poly-policies phenomenon discussed in Chapter 3.

Lobbying becomes especially intense when some target/interest groups strongly support, while others oppose, the formulation of a particular policy or the manner in which it is implemented. To illustrate, some of the various groups' preferences for the results of health reform legislation are listed in Figure 4.2. While there are some similarities among the preferences of the various groups, there are also some important differences. Policymakers generally can anticipate that these groups will seek to have their preferences reflected in any policies that are enacted and to have them influence the subsequent implementation of such policies as well.

Meeting all the preferences of some target/interest groups will conflict with the preferences of other groups. Policymakers almost always face this dilemma when they confront important choices in the formulation and implementation of policies. As was noted in Chapter 2, in such situations legislators can be expected to seek to maximize their *net* political support through their decisions and actions. The same can be said for those responsible for the managment of implementing agencies and organizations. This means that rulemaking will often be influenced by interest groups' wishes and preferences, with the more powerful interests exerting the greatest influence.

Health policy in the United States, at both federal and state levels, is replete with examples of the influence of interest groups in the rulemaking stage. One such example can be seen in the rulemaking that stemmed from the enactment of the Medicare program. In part to improve its chances for passage, the Medicare legislation (P.L. 89-97) was written so that the Social Security Administration (the original implementing agency, subsequently replaced by the Health Care Financing Administration) would reimburse hospitals and physicians in their customary manner. This meant a policy of fee-for-service payments, with the fees established by the providers. Each time providers gave services to Medicare program beneficiaries, the providers were paid their "usual and customary" fees.

Figure 4.2   Target Group Preferences for Results of Health Reform

Federal Government
- Deficit reduction
- Control over growth of Medicare and Medicaid costs
- Fewer uninsured citizens
- Slower growth in health care costs

State Government
- Medicaid funding relief
- More Medicaid flexibility
- Fewer uninsured citizens
- More federal funds and slower growth in health care costs

Employers
- Slower growth in health care costs
- Simplified benefit administration
- Elimination of cost-shifting

Consumers
- Insurance availability
- Access to care (with choices)
- Lower deductibles and copays

Insurers
- Administrative simplification
- Elimination of cost-shifting
- Slower growth in health care costs

Technology Producers
- Continued demand
- Sustained research funding
- Favorable tax treatment

Individual Practitioners
- Income maintenance
- Professional autonomy
- Malpractice reform

Provider Organizations
- Improved financial condition
- Administrative simplification
- Less uncompensated care

Suppliers
- Continued demand
- Sustained profitability

Professional Schools
- Continued demand
- Student subsidies

However, some prepaid providers, such as health maintenance organizations, had a different method of charging for their services. Their approach was to charge an annual fee per patient no matter how many times the patient might see a physician or use a hospital. In this situation, the hospitals and fee-for-service physicians had an obvious preference for having the Social Security Administration reimburse them according to their customary payment pattern. But, in addition they could see an advantage in not permitting the competing prepaid organizations to be paid in their customary manner—that is, in making them subject to the fee-for-service payment rules. Their preferences, vigorously made known to the Social Security Administration through the American Medical Association and to a somewhat lesser extent through the American Hospital Association, resulted in the prepaid organizations being forced to operate under fee-for-service payment rules until the rules were finally changed in 1985 (Feldstein 1988).

After laws or programs are enacted, and after initial rules necessary for implementing them have been promulgated, the implementation phase enters a policy operation stage (see Figure 4.1). In this stage, those involved in policy implementation seek to fulfill the mandates inherent in the laws they are responsible for implementing, and to do so by following the rules and regulations promulgated to guide implementation. As we will see in the next section, however, there is always the possibility that some individuals with implementing responsibilities will disagree with the purposes of enacted laws and will seek to stall, alter, or even subvert the laws in their implementation phases. The power of those with implementation responsibilities to affect the final outcomes and consequences of policies should not be underestimated. It is a similar power to that possessed by those with operational responsibilities in private sector organizations over the achievement of organizational missions and objectives.

Policy Operation

The policy operation stage of implementation (see Figure 4.1) involves the actual running of programs and activities embedded in enacted legislation. This stage is the domain, although not exclusively, of the appointees and civil servants who staff the government. Two variables are especially important to the successful operation of policies: the policies themselves and the characteristics and capabilities of the organizations charged with their implementation. Each of these variables is examined.

The impact of the policies themselves on their implementation

As with any writing that is intended to influence the actions, behaviors, or decisions of others (e.g., legal contracts or procedure manuals), the language and construction of an individual policy plays a crucial role in the course and success of its implementation. The impact of the construction of a policy can be felt in both the rulemaking and policy operating stages. Well-written policies begin with clearly articulated goals, although clear goals are only part of what makes a good policy.

When the goals of a policy are not clear or when there are multiple or conflicting goals for a policy, successful implementation is made more difficult, if not impossible, even before the effort begins. An example of this problem can be found in the National Health Planning and Resources Development Act of 1974 (P.L. 93-641). Errantly, Congress hoped this policy would fulfill the bulk of objectives it had attempted to attain through a wide variety of earlier, more focused policies (Longest 1988). As outlined in Section 1513 of P.L. 93-641, its multiple objectives included:

- Improving the health of residents of a health service area
- Increasing the accessibility (including overcoming geographic, architectural, and transportation barriers), acceptability, continuity, and quality of health care services
- Restraining increases in the cost of providing services.

One person, commenting on the multiple goals embedded in P.L. 93-641, has correctly observed that "the legislation proposed every health system desideratum its authors could imagine" (Morone 1990, 272). The expansive set of inherently contradictory goals eventually doomed the policy; Congress repealed P.L. 93-641 in 1986.

Vague or conflicting goals are not the only potentially serious problems with the construction of policies—problems that can make implementation very difficult if not impossible. The procedural paradigm set forth in a policy can also be flawed. Embedded in every policy is a hypothesis: "if a, b, c, and so on, are done at time one, then x, y, z, and so on will result at time two" (Thompson 1991, 151). The causal relationship implied in the construction of policies reflects that policies themselves are but means to ends—the ends being the solution of problems.

If the hypothesis embedded in a policy is wrong, the policy cannot be effectively implemented because the policy will not solve the problem it is intended to address. It will not matter that its goals are appropriate, or even that they are noble. In creating the National Health Planning and Resources Development Act, for example, Congress patched together an odd pair of conceptual ideas: voluntary, community-based planning on the one hand, and heavy-handed regulation, at least of capital expansion in the health sector, on the other. To no one's surprise, at least in hindsight, the combination did not work very well. The core hypothesis of the policy was flawed.

Another potential difficulty with the construction of policies is the nature and extent of decisions left to the implementing agencies by virtue of explicitly directive language in a statute, by what is not said in a statute, or by confusing or vague language in a statute. While a degree of flexibility in developing the rules and regulations to be used in policy implementation can be advantageous, vague directives included in policies can create all sorts of problems for those with implementation responsibilities. The 30 pages of the Occupational Safety and Health Act of 1970 (P.L. 91-596), for example, contained a number of vague directives and phrases that gave its implementors significant problems. It also contained some very explicit directives that also gave the implementors difficulty.

In Section 2 of the statute, the language stressed the importance of fostering healthful working conditions "so far as possible." This language was in lieu of specific objectives or targets for achieving reductions in occupational injuries or diseases. In Section 6, the statute authorized the secretary of labor, in implementing the law, to promulgate standards dealing with toxic substances in the workplace "to the extent feasible." In the implementation phase, considerable time and energy were expended in attempting to decide whether this phrase meant that implementors could take the economic costs of their actions to employers into account in establishing standards dealing with toxic substances. In these instances, effective implementation was impeded by some of the policy's vague and imprecise language.

In combination with such imprecise language as that noted above, Congress was surprisingly precise in writing into the law the range of fines that could be assessed against firms that violated standards. For less serious violations, the fine would be $1,000. For serious, willful violations, the fine could be up to $10,000. Most analysts considered the limits of these fines to be far too low to be effective deterents, especially for large, profitable enterprises. In this instance, effective implementation was impeded by specific language contained in the policy.

The impact of implementing organizations on policy implementation

One important constant in the dynamic circumstances that are involved in the implementation of policies is that the bulk of the implementation responsibility rests in executive branch organizational units. HCFA is primarily responsible for implementing the Medicare program; the Food and Drug Administration is primarily responsible for implementing many of the nation's food and drug policies. State insurance departments are responsible for implementing the states' policies regarding health insurance, and so on. The essence of the implementation phase of policymaking is that one or more organizations or agencies take actions that are designed to implement the intent of the legislatures that enact policies.

Since implementation responsibilities rest so heavily with executive branch agencies and organizations, all of which fall under the authority of the chief executive, it is easy to ascribe more coordination and coherence to the manner in which these responsibilities are discharged than is generally warranted, especially in the case of the huge and complex federal bureaucracy. The roles of the federal agencies most involved in the implementation of the nation's policies regarding pesticides in the food supply provide a good illustrative example of some of the problems that exist in the implementation of policies.

Although the Clinton administration has vowed to change this situation and is taking concrete steps to do so, the nation's performance on this important aspect of environmental safety has been frought with problems. Three federal agencies are heavily involved in implementing the nation's pesticide policies. Traditionally, the Environmental Protection Agency (EPA) has been responsible for testing for pesticide residue in the food supply; the Food and Drug Administration (FDA) has been responsible for analyzing the safety of pesticide products; and the U.S. Department of Agriculture has worked to keep pesticides on the market to boost farm production and incomes.

Acknowledging that past policies and their disjointed implementation have not adequately protected the citizenry, especially children, from pesticides in the food supply, these three agencies have adopted a new shared goal: to give a higher priority to protecting people against pesticides in food and to removing those pesticides that pose the greatest risk from the market (Burros 1993). And they have publicly committed themselves to a coordinated effort to achieve this goal. It remains to be seen if this new implementation strategy will be an improvement, and if so, whether it will become a model for other implementing organizations to emulate in carrying out their responsibilities.

After a basic organizational model of the structure of implementing organizations is presented in the next section, several of the characteristics that seem most important in determining an organization's degree of success in implementing policies are considered. Prominent among these characteristics is the ability of organizations to work cooperatively in interorganizational efforts.

The structure of implementing organizations

Organizations, whether they are in the private sector or the public sector, and whether they are relatively simple enterprises or large bureaucracies, have five interrelated parts. Mintzberg (1979, 1981, 1983) labels them the strategic apex, the operating core, the middle line, the technostructure, and the support staff.

- *The strategic apex* is comprised of those people who establish the strategic direction of an organization. In the government organizations responsible for policy implementation, this apex includes the chief executive (president, governor, mayor) and top officials such as cabinet secretaries and agency directors.
- *The operating core* are those who do the basic work of the organization. In HCFA, for example, this includes the people who are directly involved in making certain that Medicare-eligible citizens are enrolled in the program, receive the benefits that they are entitled to in a quality manner, and that the service providers are properly reimbursed for their work. In the FDA, the operating

core includes those people who are directly involved in ensuring the safety of food, drugs, medical devices, biologics, cosmetics, and radiation-emitting equipment; for proper labeling and product information; and for approval of all new drugs for marketing.

- *The middle line* are managers located between the executives in the strategic apex and people in the operating core. They are the middle of the organization's chain of command. Included are department heads and heads of other units and subdivisions.

- *The technostructure* consists of staff members who help plan and control the basic work of the organization. The people in the technostructure affect the work of others. The primary role of people in the technostructure is to help standardize work. They are removed from direct operations—from the operating work flow—but "they may design it, plan it, change it, or train the people who do it" (Mintzberg 1979, 29). The technostructure in implementing organizations might include industrial engineers, risk managers, and those who support efforts for continuous quality improvement (CQI) because they help standardize work processes. It can also include strategic planners, budget analysts, and accountants who help standardize work outputs, and people who recruit and train workers because they help standardize the skills available in the organization's workforce.

- *Support staff* provide indirect services. In Mintzberg's conceptualization, they provide support to the organization's basic work, but do not do the basic work. In implementing organizations, support staff might include people involved in media relations, in legislative relations, legal counsel, public relations, finance, and human resources management. Support staff differ from people in the technostructure primarily in that support staff do not focus on work standardization. Support staff provide services to the organization that permit it do its basic work.

The five parts of many implementing organizations can be diagrammed as shown in Figure 4.3. This structure

> shows a small strategic apex connected by a flaring middle line to a large, flat operating core. These three parts of the organization are shown in one uninterrupted sequence to indicate that they are typically connected through a single line of formal authority. The technostructure and the support staff are shown off to either side to indicate that they are separate from this main line of authority, and influence the operating core only indirectly. (Mintzberg 1979, 20)

Mintzberg labels such an organization a *machine bureaucracy*. Machine bureaucracies are characterized by large, well-developed techno-

Figure 4.3   Mintzberg's Machine Bureaucracy

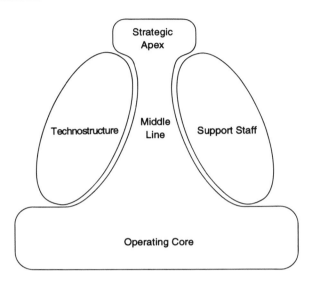

From Henry Mintzberg, *The Structuring of Organizations,* © 1979, p. 20. Reprinted by permission of Prentice-Hall, Englewood Cliffs, New Jersey.

structures and support staffs because there is great emphasis on work standardization and a focus on maintaining good relationships with the legislative branch and with the media as well as on maintaining strong financial and operational control systems in machine bureaucracies. Major decisions are made in the strategic apex, which features rigid patterns of authority. Spans of control are narrow, decision making is centralized, and the organization is functionally departmentalized. This design, which is characteristic of many government agencies and units, can also be found in the private sector, especially in large manufacturing organizations.

Figure 4.4 depicts an important variation on the machine bureaucracy, which Mintzberg has labeled the *professional bureaucracy.* The professional bureaucracy is characterized by an operating core composed primarily of professionals. This design is found in some implementing organizations such as the Centers for Disease Control, FDA, Justice Department, and the National Institutes of Health—organizations that are dominated by professionals. In the private sector, the professional bureaucracy form can be found in such organizations as teaching hospitals, law firms, and public accounting firms.

Figure 4.4   Mintzberg's Professional Bureaucracy

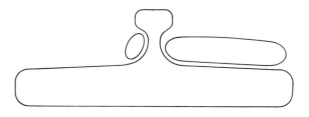

From Henry Mintzberg, *The Structuring of Organizations*, © 1979, p. 355. Reprinted by permission of Prentice-Hall, Englewood Cliffs, New Jersey.

In the professional bureaucracy, the operating core is the heart of the organization and more decision making is decentralized to it. The technostructure is underdeveloped because work is largely done by professionals who do not need—indeed, do not permit—others to heavily influence their work. In larger professional bureaucracies, support staff may be highly developed and diverse because this staff is needed to support the professionalized operating core.

Characteristics of successful implementing organizations

Several characteristics of implementing organizations are relevant to their abilities to successfully implement health policies. Among the most important are the fit between the implementing organizations and the purposes and goals of the policies they are charged to implement; the quality of the implementing organizations' leadership; the ability of implementing organizations to work smoothly with other organizations that are involved in implementation; and the appropriateness of the technologies for implementation that are available in the implementing organizations (Morone 1992). Each of these characteristics is important to the ability of an implementing organization to succeed in its task of implementing policies.

The fit between implementing organizations and the goals of the policies they seek to implement. No characteristic of an implementing organization is more basic to success than a close fit between the organization and the purposes and goals of the policies it must implement. According to Morone (1992), the keys here include whether or not the organization is sympathetic to the policy's goals and whether or not the organization has the necessary resources (i.e., money, personnel, prestige, and skills) to effectively implement the policy.

Especially important among the needed skills are those of the implementing organization's leadership. Necessary support for the implementation task must be garnered, and the policy and its implementation must be protected from unwarranted amendments or intrusions by those who do not support the policy. Allies in the legislative branch and among interest groups can be very important to this process, but much of the responsibility rests with the leaders of the implementing organization.

The quality of the implementing organizations' leadership. The manner in which the directors and managers of implementing organizations (the people in the strategic apex) play their organizational leadership roles directly affect the performance levels achieved in policy implementation. As organization leaders, these people face demanding responsibilities, such as:

- Molding a widely shared internal *and* external agreement on the implementing organization's purposes and priorities
- Building widespread support for the organization's purposes and priorities among internal and external stakeholders, especially among legislative overseers and relevant interest groups
- Striking a workable balance among the economic and professional interests of the organization's members, its external stakeholders, and the public interest the organization is required to serve
- Negotiating and maintaining effective relationships with other people and/or organizations who are regulated or otherwise affected by the implementing organization, who supply resources to the implementing organization, and with other organizations with whom the implementing organization must work closely in carrying out its policy implementation role.

The fulfillment of these responsibilities requires that the leaders of implementing organizations engage in transformational leadership (Burns 1978). It also requires that they be adept at conflict management and negotiation (Polzer and Neale 1994) and at communication (Longest and Klingensmith 1994). Although intensive attention to the role of leadership in transforming or revitalizing organizations is a recent phenomenon (Bass 1985), it is what people often mean when they speak of leadership. When an implementing organization or agency is perceived as successful because of "good leadership," this generally means that leadership decisions such as those regarding organizational mission and structure, priorities, quality standards, and the acquisition of new technologies have been good decisions, not just that the organization's managers have summoned extra motivation and performance from organization members, or helped plan their tasks, or taught them new skills. These latter activities are important to an implementing organization's success. They are generally known as transactional leadership in that the leader enters into a transaction with followers in which certain needs of the followers are met if they perform to the leader's expectations (Burns 1978). But such transactions are not the main determinants of the success of those who lead policy implementing organizations. In this role, the focus must be on leadership of the entire organization, and here the game is transformational leadership.

The essence of transformational leadership is the ability to develop and instill in members of the organization a common vision and to stimulate determined adherence to that vision. Leaders at the organizational level must focus on the various decisions and activities that affect the entire organization, including those intended to ensure its survival and overall health. In effect, their role is to "manage culture" (McLaughlin and Kaluzny 1990).

Organizational leaders must also establish goals; inculcate certain values in the organization; build intra- and interorganizational coalitions; and interpret and respond to various challenges and opportunities presented to the organization from its external environment, which includes taking steps necessary to alter the constraints placed on the organization by its external environment when necessary.

Organizational leadership is directly affected by the context in which it takes place. For example, organizational leadership is facilitated in implementing organizations where

- The existence of longstanding shared values and commonly accepted principles help shape the organization's mission and operating practices and resolve conflicts among competing views
- A history of successfully implementing policies helps legitimatize the organization's claims for support from internal and external stakeholders
- The technical ability to do good strategic planning, develop effective relationships with oversight actors and relevant interest groups, and the availability of adequate financial resources provide a sense of organizational pride, stability, and an appropriate degree of self-determination and autonomy.

Organizational leadership is also affected by other management skills—most notably, communication and motivation skills. Leaders who can effectively articulate and communicate their visions will have a distinct advantage in having them considered and in providing guidance for the behaviors of their followers. While we have long recognized the relationship between strategic vision and effective leadership, we have only recently begun to understand the critical link between the leader's ability to effectively communicate the vision and success. It is now quite clear that the best organizational leaders are not only effective strategists and visionaries, but effective communicators as well (Conger 1991). Furthermore, successful organizational leaders must be able to mobilize widespread commitment among followers to their vision for the organization and motivate the contributions of followers to the realization of the vision.

Interorganizational relationships and capabilities. When more than one organization is involved in the implementation of a policy, as is frequently the case, the nature of the interorganizational relationships that have been previously established and the general capabilities of the implementing organization to work effectively with other organizations that it must participate with in carrying out its implementation responsibilities become important issues. Rarely is a health policy implemented by a single organization or agency, and never when the policy is large in scope. Implementation of the Medicaid program, for example, involves the federal HCFA working with the Medicaid agencies in each state and with such private sector organizations as hospitals and nursing homes. The successful implementation of the Medicaid program depends heavily on the quality of the interactions among these and other organizations. The responsibility does not simply rest with a single organization.

There are two crucial managerial capabilities needed in establishing efficacious and efficient interorganizational relationships. First, skill in discerning the necessity for developing such linkages is needed. Second, skill at choosing from a menu of possible linking mechanisms those most appropriate for each situation is needed (Longest 1990). In applying these skills, managers must realize that not all interorganizational relationships used in support of policy implementation are of equal importance. Some relationships have long-term strategic purposes and some do not. The ability to discern between them is critical in allocating time and other resources that go into establishing and maintaining these relationships.

Interorganizational relationships that are of relatively more strategic importance, in terms of their impact on the outcome of implementation, and those that are relatively more permanent, or at least those intended to be permanent in terms of future shared implementation responsibilities, obviously require more attention than those of less strategic importance or those not expected to be long-term or permanent.

In making judgments about which interorganizational relationships to devote resources to establishing, it is useful for those with implementing responsibilities to remember that there are several types of such relationships among organizations. They can be pooled, sequential, or reciprocal (Thompson 1967).

Pooled relationships involve situations in which organizations are related but do not bear a particularly close or interdependent working connection; they simply contribute separately in some way to a larger whole. For example, the Public Health Service and the Social Security Administration are both major divisions of the U.S. Department of Health and Human Services, but their interrelationships tend to be merely pooled (e.g., they both belong to the same larger organizational home). Wise managers of these organizations would neither ignore relationships with each other, nor would they devote inordinate resources to establishing and maintaining the relationships.

Sequential relationships involve situations in which organizations bear a close and sequential working connection. For example, the relationships between the central office of the U.S. Department of Health and Human Services and its regional offices are sequential. Health care providers who are affected by the implementation of a health policy through the DHHS would routinely relate to the regional office first and then to the central office, in sequence. The managers in these two parts of the DHHS must be concerned about how effectively they work together because their sequential working relationship directly affects the outcomes that are achieved. Wise managers involved in such sequential relationships devote more resources to establishing and maintaining this type than to pooled relationships.

The third type of interorganizational relationship involves reciprocity between organizations in their working relationships. *Reciprocal* relationships occur when organizations bear a close relationship and the interdependence between them is mutual. For example, HCFA must work with private sector intermediaries (such as Blue Cross plans) who make payments to providers in administering the Medicare program. The relationships between these organizations are reciprocal. Neither can perform adequately without an effective and reciprocal working relationship with the other. Wise managers, in reciprocal relationships, devote the resources necessary to ensure that these critical relationships are properly established and maintained.

Effective management of interorganizational relationships generally is more important as it moves from pooled to sequential to reciprocal forms, and the need for managerial attention to effective linkages also increases. Linkages of the sequential or reciprocal types are relatively more complex because they involve issues such as the nature of the exchange relationships between participating organizations, which organizations will have the most power, the terms of the resource transactions between them, and how shared work will be developed and divided between the organizations.

Useful interorganizational relationships are not achieved without costs. The obvious costs are the time, personnel, and money needed to support the various relationships. There also is the potential loss of some degree of autonomy when interorganizational relationships are involved in decisions and actions. However, the benefits of establishing and maintaining appropriate and effective interorganizational relationships far outweigh the associated costs.

The organizations' repertoire of tools, methods, and technologies. Implementing organizations rely on a variety of tools, methods, and technologies to implement policies. Just as policies differ in substantial ways (remember the distinction between allocative and regulatory policies made in Chapter 1), the technologies needed to implement them also differ (Thompson 1991).

Regulatory polices require such technologies as those through which implementing organizations prescribe and control the behaviors of one or more target groups. These technologies include rule promulgation, investigatory capacity, and the ability to impose sanctions. Allocative policies require technologies such as those through which implementing organizations deliver income, goods, or services. Technologies of this type include targeting recipients or beneficiaries, determining eligibility for benefits, and managing the supply and quality of goods or services provided through the policy.

The Occupational Safety and Health Administration, for example, relies heavily on regulatory technologies as it seeks to protect workers from hazards in the workplace. In contrast, HCFA relies heavily, although not exclusively, on allocative technologies in implementing the Medicare program.

The cyclical relationship between rulemaking and policy operation

A close examination of the implementation phase depicted in Figure 4.1 reveals that rulemaking precedes policy operation, but that the operational activities feed back into rulemaking. This cyclical relationship is quite important. It means that experience gained with the operation of policies can influence the modification of rules and regulations used in the implementation phase. Practically, this means that the rules and regulations promulgated to implement policies can undergo revision—sometimes the revision is extensive and continuous—and that new rules can be adopted as experience dictates. This feature of policymaking tends to make the process much more dynamic than it would otherwise be.

Conclusion

The policy implementation phase of policymaking involves rulemaking and policy operation. Rulemaking is a necessary part of policymaking because enacted legislation seldom contains enough explicit and directive language concerning how the legislation is to be implemented to completely guide the implementation process. Routinely, implementing organizations must promulgate rules to guide the operation of enacted policies. The promulgation of rules is itself guided by certain rules and established procedures. These help ensure that those who will be affected by the implementation of a policy have ample opportunity to participate in the rulemaking associated with its implementation.

The second set of activities in the implementation phase of policymaking involves the actual running of the programs embedded in enacted legislation. These activities are termed policy operation and are largely the domain of the appointees and civil servants who staff the government. Two variables that are quite important to the successful operation of policies are examined in this chapter. First, policies themselves, especially the language expressing the goals or objectives of the policies, have a direct impact on their implementation. Related to this, the level of flexibility permitted the implementing organizations, directly affect the course of implementation and the outcome for any policy. A second variable that heavily influences the implementation experience with any policy is the set of characteristics and capabilities of the organizations charged with its implementation.

The middle section of Figure 4.1, where the policy formulation phase bridges to the policy implementation phase, has a linear simplicity. Policy is formulated and then it is implemented. As the figure illustrates, changing biological, cultural, demographic, ecological, economic, ethical, psychological, social, and technological circumstances constantly stimulate the need to amend existing policies or establish new ones. Such changes are made legislatively and the resulting policies are implemented. But, as the figure also illustrates, shifts in the external inputs are not the only forces for change in the policymaking process.

The process includes internal features that stimulate changes in policies. The policy modification phase of the process, which is shown as a feedback loop in the model, brings the process full circle and emphasizes one of its most important features. The operational experiences gained in implementing policies and the outcomes, perceptions, and consequences of implementing existing policies also trigger policy modification. The modification phase of policymaking is explored more fully in the next chapter.

References

Bass, B. M. *Leadership and Performance Beyond Expectations*. New York: Academic Press, 1985.

Burns, J. M. *Leadership*. New York: Harper & Row, 1978.

Burros, M. "U.S. Is Taking Aim at Farm Chemicals in the Food Supply." *The New York Times*, 27 June 1993.

Conger, J. A. "Inspiring Others: The Language of Leadership." *The Executive* 5, no. 1 (February 1991): 31–45.

Feldstein, P. J. *The Politics of Health Legislation: An Economic Perspective*. Ann Arbor, MI: Health Administration Press, 1988.

Iglehart, J. K. "The American Health Care System: Medicare." *New England Journal of Medicine* 327, no. 20 (12 November 1992) 1467–72.

Longest, B. B., Jr. "American Health Policy in the Year 2000." *Hospital & Health Services Administration* 33, no. 4 (Winter 1988): 419–34.

——. "Interorganizational Linkages in the Health Sector." *Health Care Management Review* 15, no. 1 (Winter 1990): 17–28.

Longest, B. B., Jr., and J. M. Klingensmith. "Coordination and Communication." In *Health Care Management: Organization Design and Behavior*, 3d ed., edited by S. M. Shortell and A. D. Kaluzny, 182–211. Albany, NY: Delmar Publishers Inc., 1994.

McLaughlin, C. P., and A. D. Kaluzny. "Total Quality Management in Health: Making it Work." *Health Care Management Review* 15, no. 3 (Summer 1990): 7–14.

Mintzberg, H. "Organizational Design: Fashion or Fit?" *Harvard Business Review* 59, no. 1 (January–February 1981): 103–16.

——. *Structure in Fives: Designing Effective Organizations*. Englewood Cliffs, NJ: Prentice-Hall, 1983.

——. *The Structuring of Organizations*. Englewood Cliffs, NJ: Prentice-Hall, 1979.

Morone, J. A. "Administrative Agencies and the Implementation of National Health Care Reform." In *Implementation Issues and National Health Care Reform*, edited by C. Brecher, 47–72. Proceedings of a conference sponsored by the Robert F. Wagner Graduate School of Public Service, New York University, June 1992.

——. *The Democratic Wish: Popular Participation and the Limits of American Government*. New York: Basic Books, 1990.

Polzer, J. T., and M. A. Neale. "Conflict Management and Negotiation." In *Health Care Management: Organization Design and Behavior*, 3d ed., edited by S. M. Shortell and A. D. Kaluzny, 113–33. Albany, NY: Delmar Publishers Inc., 1994.

Rakich, J. S., B. B. Longest, Jr., and K. Darr. *Managing Health Services Organizations*, 3d ed. Baltimore, MD: Health Professions Press, 1992. (See especially Chapters 12 and 16.)

Thompson, F. J. "The Enduring Challenge of Health Policy Implementation." In

Health Politics and Policy, 2d ed., edited by T. J. Litman and L. S. Robins, 148–69. Albany, NY: Delmar Publishers Inc., 1991.

Thompson, J. D. *Organizations in Action*. New York: McGraw-Hill, 1967.

Zwick, D. I. "Initial Development of Guidelines for Health Planning." *Public Health Reports* 93 (1978): 407–20.

Figure 5.1 A Model of the Public Policymaking Process in the United States: The Policy Modification Phase

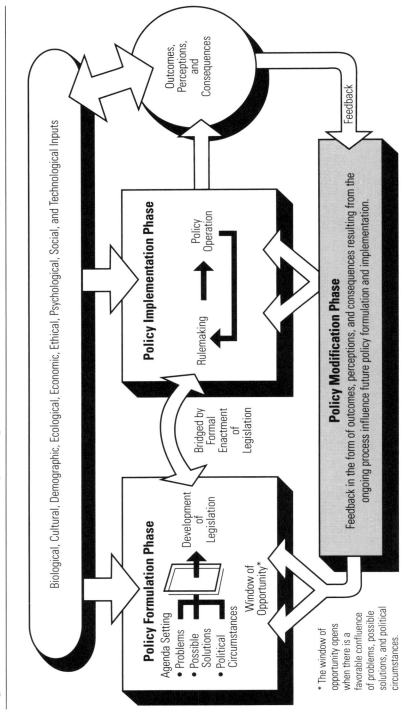

5

Policy Modification

This chapter addresses the policy modification phase of public policymaking (see the shaded portion of Figure 5.1). Conceptually, policy modification can be separated from policy initiation although in reality the two are closely intertwined. Policy initiation results when the confluence of problems, possible solutions, and political circumstances lead to the *initial* development of legislation in the formulation phase (as was described in Chapter 3) and then to subsequent rulemaking and policy operation as the policy is implemented, as was described in Chapter 4. Policy modification, in contrast to initiation, results when the outcomes, perceptions, and consequences of existing policies feed back into the agenda-setting and legislation-development stages of the formulation phase and into the rulemaking and policy operation stages of the implementation phase and stimulate *changes* in legislation, rules, or operations. This is shown as the feedback loop in Figure 5.1.

The history of American health policy shows clearly that we can, and on occasion do, initiate new policies. For example, in 1798 the Congress established the U.S. Marine Hospital Service to provide medical care for sick and disabled seamen. This was the initial policy from which eventually grew the U.S. Public Health Service. In 1921 Congress enacted the initial Maternity and Infancy Act (P.L. 67-97) through which grants were made to states to encourage them to develop health services for mothers and children. This new policy became the prototype for federal grants-in-aid to the states. In 1935 Congress enacted the Social Security Act (P.L. 74-271), which initiated the major entrance of the federal government into the area of social insurance. This policy now encompasses, among many other things, the Medicare and Medicaid programs.

These examples show that some health policies are indeed developed de novo. But a very important feature of health policymaking in the United States is that the vast majority of contemporary health policies spring from a relatively few early initial policies. Most health policies are the result of modifying prior policies, which is why understanding the modification phase of the process is so important. A review of the chronology of important American health policies, such as the one contained in the Appendix, readily illustrates just how frequently enacted health policies are but amendments of previously enacted legislation.

In fact, so many of the public policies developed through the cyclical process pictured in Figure 5.1 result from the modification of existing policies, and so many of the modifications represent only modest changes, that the entire public policymaking process in the United States has been characterized as a process of *incrementalism* (Lindblom 1959). In this conceptualization of policymaking, significant departures from the existing patterns of policies occur only rarely.

The process of incrementalism (the building on existing policies by modification in small incremental steps) provides a mechanism for compromises to be reached among diverse interests. For some people, words like incrementalism and compromise in policymaking conjure up a negative image, featuring such things as compromised principles, inappropriate influence peddling, and corrupt deals made behind closed doors. But, positively, "In a democracy compromise is not merely unavoidable; it is a source of creative invention, sometimes generating solutions that unexpectedly combine seemingly opposed ideas" (Starr and Zelman 1993, 8).

The major participants in the policymaking process (i.e., policymakers in all three branches of government as well as most organized interest groups) have a preference for incrementalism in policymaking. This is certainly the case for most members of the health policy community. The primary reason for this preference is that the results and consequences of incrementally made decisions are more predictable and stable than is the case with less incrementally made decisions.

National health policy is replete with examples of patterns of incrementally developed policies. For instance, the history of the evolution of the National Institutes of Health (NIH) vividly reflects incremental policymaking over a span of more than 50 years. Beginning in the 1930s as a small federal laboratory conducting biomedical research, the NIH has experienced extensive elaboration (the addition of new institutes as biomedical science evolved), growth (its annual budget is now more than $10 billion), and shifts in the emphases of its research agenda (cancer, AIDS, women's health, etc.). Every step in its continuing evolution has been guided by specific changes in policies, each one an incremental modification intended to have the NIH make only marginal adjustments in its actions, decisions, and behaviors.

The Modification Phase

As the feedback arrows contained in Figure 5.1 illustrate, policies can be modified at four points in the policymaking process: in the (1) agenda-setting and (2) legislation-development stages of the formulation phase and in the (3) rulemaking and (4) policy operation stages of the implementation phase.

The policymaking process provides abundant opportunities for the outcomes, perceptions, and consequences that result from the implementation of policies to influence the reformulation of policies, either through influencing agenda setting or through the amendment of prior legislation. The amendment of prior legislation occurs through the process of legislation development just as does the creation of an entirely new legislative proposal. The only significant difference is that the possibility of amendment implies the existence of a particular prior piece of legislation that can be changed. This prior legislation already has a developmental history and an implementation experience, both of which can influence its amendment.

As we will explore more fully in the next section, using the Medicare program as an example, health policies are routinely amended, some of them repeatedly and over a span of many years. Such amendments reflect, among other things, the emergence of new medical technologies, changing federal budgetary conditions, and beneficiary demands. These and other stimuli for change often gain the attention of policymakers through the routine activities and reporting mechanisms that occur in implementing existing policies. Modification of prior policies is an integral part of health policy formulation in the United States.

Feedback about the outcomes, perceptions, and consequences resulting from the implementation of policies can also stimulate the modification of policies in the implementation phase. The results of policy implementation routinely lead to modifications in the rulemaking and policy operation stages, and often in both concurrently. Such adjustments are directed by the managers of the implementing organizations and are like the activities that managers of all sorts of activities engage in when they seek to control the results of their operations. Standards or operating objectives are established, operations ensue, results are monitored, and changes are made in operations or objectives, or both, when results do not measure up to the predetermined standards. Such routine operational modifications are inherent in the implementation phase of any policy. They are part of the daily work that occurs within organizations that implement health policies.

In the following sections, we will explore each of these paths to the modification of health policies, beginning with the impact of modification on agenda setting and legislation development.

Modification in the Formulation Phase

The outcomes, perceptions, and consequences of the ongoing policymaking cycle can readily influence the modification of health policies by directly and forcefully affecting the agenda-setting stage of the cycle.

Modification at the agenda-setting stage

Remember that agenda setting involves the confluence of problems, possible solutions, and political circumstances. Policy modification can occur at this stage as problems become more sharply defined and better understood within the context of ongoing implementation of existing policies. Possible solutions to problems can be assessed and clarified within the same context, especially when operational experience and the results of demonstrations and evaluations provide concrete evidence of the performance of particular solutions that are under consideration. And the interactions among the branches of government and interest groups involved with and affected by ongoing policies become important components of the political circumstances surrounding their reformulation, as well as of the initial formulation of future policies.

Modification at the legislation-development stage

The outcomes, perceptions, and consequences that flow from the ongoing policymaking process also help modify policies by directly influencing the development of legislation. This very common occurrence reflects the fact that the operational experience with the implementation of policies can help identify needed modifications in their underlying legislation.

In addition, certain policies—such as those intended to reduce the federal budget deficit—can and do impinge on other policies, often causing their modification. For example, implementation of the Deficit Reduction Act of 1984 (P.L. 98-369) required a temporary freeze on physicians' fees paid under the Medicare program; and implementation of the Emergency Deficit Reduction and Balanced Budget Act of 1985 (P.L. 99-177), also known as the Gramm-Rudman-Hollins Act, required budget cuts in defense and in certain domestic programs including a number of health programs.

Examples of modification in the formulation phase

The phenomenon of policy modification, in both the agenda-setting and legislation-development stages, is vividly reflected in the legislative history of the development of the Medicare program. The abbreviated chronology of the legislation related to this program that follows provides a background for considering some of the ways in which the modification phase of policymaking alters policies in the formulation phase.

An abbreviated legislative history of the Medicare program

1935: Social Security Act (P.L. 74-271). This landmark legislation, enacted during the Great Depression, began the expansion of the federal government's central role in the domain of social insurance. Importantly for the future of federal health policy, it included provisions through which the federal government made grants-in-aid to states for the support of programs for the needy elderly, dependent children, and the blind. Over the years, a number of amendments were made to the act, including the amendments of 1960 (P.L. 86-778), known as the Kerr-Mills Act, which established a new program for medical assistance for the aged.

1965: Social Security Amendments of 1965 (P.L. 89-97). This legislation provided health insurance for the aged through Title 18 (Medicare) and provided grants to the states for medical assistance programs for the poor through Title 19 (Medicaid). (These programs are described in more detail in Note 1 in Chapter 1 and in the chronology of federal laws presented in the Appendix.)

Part A of Medicare provided hospital insurance benefits intended to protect beneficiaries against certain costs of hospital and related post-hospital services. These benefits were financed by an increase in the Social Security earnings tax (payroll tax). Part B of Medicare provided supplemental medical insurance benefits intended to protect beneficiaries from the costs of certain physician services, laboratory tests, supplies, and equipment, as well as certain home health services. These benefits were financed by voluntary premium payments from those who chose to enroll, matched by payments from general revenues.[1]

1967: Social Security Amendments of 1967 (P.L. 90-248). The first modifications, coming two years after the Medicare program's establishment, featured expanded coverage for such things as durable medical equipment for use in the home, podiatrist services for nonroutine foot care and outpatient physical therapy under Part B, and the addition of a lifetime reserve of 60 days of coverage for inpatient hospital care over and above the original coverage for up to 90 days during any spell of illness. In addition, certain payment rules were modified in favor of providers. For example, payment of full reasonable charges for radiologists' and pathologists' services provided to inpatients were authorized under one modification.

1972: Social Security Amendments of 1972 (P.L. 92-603). Although, in part, they continued the pattern of program expansions started in the 1967 modifications, these amendments marked an important shift to some policy modifications that were intended specifically to help control the growing costs of the Medicare program. Among the most important of the 1972 modifications was the establishment of Professional Standards Review Organizations (PSROs), which were to monitor both the quality of services provided to Medicare beneficiaries as well as the medical necessity for the services.

Another modification aimed at cost containment was the addition of a provision to limit payments for capital expenditures by hospitals that had been disapproved by state or local planning agencies. Still another was the authorization of grants and contracts to conduct experiments and demonstrations related to achieving increased economy and efficiency in the provision of health services. Some of the specifically targeted areas of these studies were to be prospective reimbursement, the requirement that patients spend three days in the hospital prior to admission to a skilled nursing home, the potential benefits of ambulatory surgery centers, payment for the services of physician's assistants and nurse practitioners, and the use of clinical psychologists.

At the same time that these and other cost-containment modifications were made in the Medicare policy, a number of cost-increasing changes were also made. Notably, persons who were eligible for cash benefits under the disability provisions of the Social Security Act for at least 24 months were made eligible for medical benefits under the Medicare program. In addition, persons who were insured under Social Security, as well as their dependents, who required hemodialysis or renal transplantation for chronic renal disease were defined as disabled for the purpose of having them covered under the Medicare program for the costs of treating their end-stage renal disease (ESRD). The inclusion of coverage for the disabled and ESRD patients in 1972 were extraordinarily expensive modifications of the Medicare program. In addition, certain less costly but still expensive additional coverages were extended, including chiropractic services and speech pathology services.

1976–1977: A major reorganization of the U.S. Department of Health, Education and Welfare (now the U.S. Department of Health and Human Services). While not technically a modification of the Medicare policy, this reorganization resulted in the establishment of the Health Care Financing Administration (HCFA) that assumed primary responsibility for implementation of the Medicare and Medicaid programs. This new agency combined functions that had been located in the Bureau of Health Insurance of the Social Security Administration (Medicare) and in the Medical Services Administration of the Social and Rehabilitation Service (Medicaid), among others.

1977: Rural Health Clinic Services Amendments (P.L. 95-210). This legislation modified the categories of practitioners who could provide reimbursable services to Medicare beneficiaries, at least in rural settings. Under the provisions of this act, rural health clinics that did not routinely have physicians available on site, could, if they met certain requirements regarding physician supervision of the clinic and review of services, be reimbursed for services provided by nurse practitioners and physician's assistants through the Medicare and Medicaid programs. This act also authorized certain demonstration projects in underserved urban areas for reimbursement of these nonphysician practitioners.

1977: Medicare-Medicaid Antifraud and Abuse Amendments (P.L. 95-142). These modifications sought to reduce fraud and abuse in both the Medicare and Medicaid programs and thereby help contain their costs. Specific changes included strengthening criminal and civil penalties for fraud and abuse affecting the programs, modification in the operations of the PSROs, and the promulgation of uniform reporting systems and formats for hospitals and certain other health care organizations participating in the Medicare and Medicaid programs.

1978: Medicare End-Stage Renal Disease Amendments (P.L. 95-292). Since the addition of coverage for ESRD under the Social Security Amendments of 1972 (P.L. 92-603), the costs to the Medicare program had risen steadily and quickly. These amendments sought to help control the program's costs. One modification added incentives to encourage the use of home dialysis and the use of renal transplantation in ESRD. Another modification permitted the use of a variety of reimbursement methods for renal dialysis facilities. Still another modification authorized studies of end-stage renal disease itself, especially studies incorporating possible cost reductions in treatment for this disease and authorized the Secretary of DHEW (now DHHS) to establish areawide network coordinating councils to help plan for and review ESRD programs.

1980: Omnibus Budget Reconciliation Act, or OBRA '80, (P.L. 96-499). Extensive modifications of Medicare and Medicaid were made in this legislation. Fifty-seven separate sections pertained to one or both of the programs. Many of the changes reflected continuing concern with the growing costs of the programs and were intended to help control these costs. Examples of the changes that were specific to Medicare included removal of the 100 visits-per-year limitation on home health services and the requirement that patients pay a deductible for home care visits under Part B of the program. These changes were intended to encourage home care over more expensive institutional care. Another provision permitted small rural hospitals to use their beds as "swing beds" (alternating their use as acute or long-term care beds as needed) and authorized swing-bed demonstration projects for large and urban hospitals.

1981: Omnibus Budget Reconciliation Act, or OBRA '81, (P.L. 97-35). Just as in 1980, this legislation included extensive changes in the Medicare and Medicaid programs (46 sections pertained to these programs). Enacted in the context of extensive efforts to make reductions in the federal budget, many of the provisons hit Medicaid especially hard, but others were aimed directly at the Medicare program. For example, one provision eliminated the coverage of alcohol detoxification facility services, another removed the use of occupational therapy as a basis for initial entitlement to home health service, and yet another increased the Part B deductible.

1982: Tax Equity and Fiscal Responsibility Act, or TEFRA, (P.L. 97-248). A number of important changes with significant impact on the Medicare program were contained in this legislation. For example, one provision added coverage for hospice services provided to Medicare beneficiaries. These benefits were extended later and are now an integral part of the Medicare program. However, the most important provisions, in terms of impact on the Medicare program, were those that sought to control the program's costs by setting limits on how much Medicare would reimburse hospitals on a per case basis and by limiting the annual rate of increase for Medicare's reasonable costs per discharge. These changes in reimbursement methodology represented fundamental changes in the Medicare program and reflected a dramatic shift in the nation's Medicare policy. Another provision of TEFRA pertained to replacing PSROs, which had been established by the Social Security Amendments of 1972 (P.L. 92-603), with a new utilization and quality control program called Peer Review Organizations (PROs). The TEFRA changes regarding the operation of the Medicare program were extensive, but they were only the harbinger of the most sweeping legislative changes in the history of the Medicare program the following year.

1983: Social Security Amendments of 1983 (P.L. 98-21). This important legislation initiated the Medicare prospective payment system (PPS) and included provisions to base payment for hospital inpatient services on predetermined rates per discharge for diagnosis-related groups (DRGs). PPS was a major departure from the cost-based system of reimbursement that had been used in the Medicare program since its inception in 1965. The dramatic impact of this change is best seen in terms of expenditures on the Medicare program. PPS reduced Medicare's hospital expenditures sharply. An analysis by Russell and Manning (1989) showed that 1990 Medicare expenditures for hospital inpatient care were approximately 20 percent lower than would have been the case without implementation of the PPS. In this act, the Congress also directed the administration to study physician payment reform options.

1984: Deficit Reduction Act, or DEFRA, (P.L. 98-369). Among the provisions of this act was one to temporarily freeze physicians' fees paid under the Medicare program. Another placed a specific limitation on the rate of increase in the DRG payment rates that the Secretary of DHHS could permit in the two subsequent years. This act also created two classes of physicians in regard to their relationships to the Medicare program and outlined different reimbursement approaches for them depending on whether they were classified as participating or nonparticipating.

1985: Emergency Deficit Reduction and Balanced Budget Act, or the Gramm-Rudman-Hollins Act, (P.L. 99-177). This legislation established mandatory deficit reduction targets for the five subsequent fiscal years. Under provisions of the law, the required budget cuts would come equally from defense spending and from domestic programs that were not exempted. The Gramm-Rudman-Hollins Act had signficant impact on the Medicare program throughout the last half of the 1980s, as well as on other health programs such as community and migrant health centers, veteran and Native American health, health professions education, and the NIH (Rhodes 1992). Among other things, this legislation led to substantial cuts in Medicare payments to hospitals and physicians.

1985: Consolidated Omnibus Budget Reconciliation Act, or COBRA '85, (P.L. 99-272). Through a number of provisions of the act that impacted on Medicare, hospitals that served a disproportionate share of poor patients received an adjustment in their PPS payments; hospice care was made a permanent part of the program; fiscal year 1986 PPS payment rates were frozen at 1985 levels through 1 May 1986 and increased 0.5 of a percent for the remainder of the year; payment to hospitals for the indirect costs of medical education were modified; and a schedule to phase out payment of a return on equity to proprietary hospitals was established.

1986: Omnibus Budget Reconciliation Act, or OBRA '86, (P.L. 99-509). This act altered the PPS payment rate for hospitals once again and reduced payment amounts for capital-related costs by 3.5 percent for part of fiscal year 1987, by 7 percent for fiscal year 1988, and by 10 percent for fiscal year 1989. In addition, certain adjustments were made in the manner in which "outlier" or atypical cases were reimbursed.

1987: Omnibus Budget Reconciliation Act, or OBRA '87 (P.L. 100-203). This legislation required the Secretary of the DHHS to update the wage index used in calculating hospital PPS payments by 1 October 1990 and to do so at least every three years thereafter. It also required the Secretary to study and report to Congress on the criteria being used by the Medicare program to identify referral hospitals. Deepening the reductions established by OBRA '86, one provision of the act reduced payment amounts for capital-related costs by 12 percent for fiscal year 1988 and 15 percent for 1989.

1988: Medicare Catastrophic Coverage Act (P.L. 100-360). This act provided the largest expansion of the benefits covered under the Medicare program since its establishment in 1965. Among other things, provisions of this act added coverage for outpatient prescription drugs and respite care and placed a cap on out-of-pocket spending for copayment costs for covered services by the elderly. The legislation included provisions that would have the new benefits phased in over a four-year period and paid for by premiums charged to Medicare program enrollees. Thirty-seven percent of the costs were to be covered by a fixed monthly premium paid by all enrollees and the remainder of the costs were to be covered by an income-related supplemental premium that was, in effect, an income tax surtax that would apply to fewer than half of the enrollees. Under intense pressure from many of their elderly constituents and their interest groups, who objected to having to pay additional premiums or the income tax surtax, Congress repealed P.L. 100-360 in 1989, without implementing most of its provisions.

1989: Omnibus Budget Reconciliation Act, or OBRA '89, (P.L. 101-239). The act included provisions for minor, primarily technical, changes in the PPS and to extend coverage for mental health benefits and add coverage for Pap smears. Small adjustments were made in the disproportionate share regulations, and the 15 percent capital-related payment reduction established in OBRA '87 was continued in OBRA '89. Another provision required the Secretary of DHHS to update the wage index annually in a budget neutral manner beginning in fiscal year 1993. The most important provision of OBRA '89 was one through which HCFA was directed to begin implementing a resource-based relative value scale (RBRVS)[2] for reimbursing physicians under the Medicare program on 1 January 1992. The new system was to be phased in over a four-year period beginning in 1992.

1990: Omnibus Budget Reconciliation Act, or OBRA '90, (P.L. 101-508). The act made additional minor changes in the PPS, including further adjustments in the wage index calculation and in the disproportionate share regulations. Regarding the wage index, one provision required ProPAC (the Prospective Payment Assessment Commission which was established by the 1983 Amendments to the Social Security Act to help guide the Congress and the Secretary of DHHS on implementing the PPS) to further study the available data on wages by occupational category and to develop recommendations on modifying the wage index to account for occupational mix. It also included a provision that continued the 15 percent capital-related payment reduction that was established in OBRA '87, and continued in OBRA '89, and another provision that made the reduced teaching adjustment payment established in OBRA '87 permanent. One of its more important provisions provided a five-year deficit reduction plan that was to reduce total Medicare outlays by more than $43 billion between fiscal years 1991 and 1995.

1993: Omnibus Budget Reconciliation Act, or OBRA '93, (P.L. 103-66). This legislation established an all-time record five-year cut in Medicare funding and included a number of other changes affecting the Medicare program. For example, the legislation included provisions to end return on equity (ROE) payments for capital to proprietary skilled nursing facilities and reduced the previously established rate of increase in payment rates for care provided in hospices. In addition, the legislation cut laboratory fees drastically by changing the reimbursement formula and froze payments for durable medical equipment, parenteral and enteral services, and for orthotics and prosthetics in fiscal years 1994 and 1995.

Annually, modifications continue to made in the Medicare program; this pattern is likely to continue as long as the program continues. Having provided some of the program's legislative history, we are now in a position to examine the pattern of policy modification reflected in that history.

The phenomenon of policy modification at work in the formulation phase

Imbedded in the chronology of Medicare-related legislation are many examples of how the policy modification phase influences the policy formulation phase. Although the chronology begins with the enactment of a new policy, the 1935 Social Security Act, it is replete with examples of how the outcomes, perceptions, and consequences associated with the implementation of a policy, in this case the Social Security Act, feed back into agenda setting and legislation development.

The Medicare program emerged on the nation's policy agenda, in large part, through the operation of the Social Security program over a span of three decades, from the mid-1930s to the mid-1960s. President Franklin D. Roosevelt formed a Committee on Economic Security in 1934 and charged its members to develop a program that could ensure the economic security of the nation's citizens. The committee considered the inclusion of health insurance as part of the social security program from the outset. There was, in fact, strong sentiment for doing so among members of the committee (Starr 1982). But in the end they decided not to recommend the inclusion of health insurance because of the political burdens associated with such a proposal. The American Medical Association, in particular, strongly opposed the concept (Peterson 1993).

As reflected in the original legislation, the Social Security Act of 1935 was:

> An Act to provide for the general welfare by establishing a system of federal old age benefits, and by enabling the several States to make more adequate provision for aged persons, blind persons, dependent and crippled children, maternal and child welfare, public health, and the administration of their unemployment compensation laws; to establish a Social Security Board; to raise revenue; and for other purposes.

Although health insurance was not included among the program's features, from time to time in the ensuing years its addition was considered. President Harry S. Truman considered national health insurance a key part of his legislative agenda (Altmeyer 1968). But the continued, powerful opposition from the American Medical Association and the necessity for the Truman administration to divert its attention to Korea in 1950 meant that President Truman was unable to stimulate the development and enactment of any sort of universal health insurance policy. Faced with dim political prospects for universal health insurance, proponents turned to a much more limited idea—hospital insurance for the aged.

Following a number of rather modest proposals for such insurance, none of which could muster the necessary political support for enactment, two powerful members of the Congress, Senator Robert Kerr (D–Okla.) and Representative Wilbur Mills (D–Ark.), were able to see through to passage a bill that provided federal support for states' programs in welfare medicine. The Amendments to the Social Security Act of 1960 (P.L. 86-778) provided health benefits to the aged, but only to the poor aged. Not until the Democratic margin in Congress was significantly increased in President Lyndon B. Johnson's landslide election in 1964 did anything more expansive have much chance of passing.

With the 1964 election significantly improving its prospects for passage, Medicare received a very high priority among President Johnson's

Great Society programs and was enacted as part of the Social Security Amendments of 1965 (P.L. 89-97). Medicare did indeed emerge on the nation's policy agenda through a series of attempts to modify the original Social Security Act by expanding the benefits provided to include health insurance.

After enactment of the Medicare program, the chronology shows a remarkable pattern of the outcomes, perceptions, and consequences associated with its implementation, feeding back into subsequent rounds of modification of the original legislation. Services were added and deleted; premiums and copayment provisions were changed; reimbursement mechanisms were changed; features to ensure quality and medical necessity of services were added, changed, and deleted; and so on.

The chronology of the Medicare program reflects significant legislative change from year to year, a pattern likely to continue as long as this complex and expensive program exists. The pattern of modifications exhibited in the Medicare legislation can be clearly seen to be heavily influenced by ongoing experience with the implementation of the original legislation and its subsequent modifications. But as we will see in the next section, not all modification of policy occurs in the formulation phase: much of it occurs in the implementation phase, where the modification process is distinctly different.

Modification in the Implementation Phase

Outcomes, perceptions, and consequences that result from the ongoing implementation of policies feed back not only to the formulation phase, but to the implementation phase as well. Modifications in this phase may occur in both the rulemaking and policy operation stages.

Modification at the rulemaking stage

As was noted in Chapter 4, rulemaking is a necessary precursor to the operation and full implementation of most policies because enacted legislation rarely contains enough explicit language describing how the legislation is to be implemented to completely guide the implementation process. Newly enacted policies are often vague on implementation details, usually purposely so, leaving it to the implementing organizations to promulgate the rules needed to guide the operation of the policies.

One of the most pervasive ways in which policies are modified is through modification of the rules and regulations used to guide their implementation. An example, again drawn from the legislative and regulatory history of the Medicare program, will help clarify this important point about how rulemaking can be used to modify policies.

An example of modification at the rulemaking stage

Among the provisions in the Social Security Amendments of 1983 (P.L. 98-213), which initiated the Medicare prospective payment system (PPS) as a means of paying hospitals based on predetermined rates per discharge for diagnosis-related groups (DRGs), was one directing the Secretary of DHHS to provide for additional payments to hospitals for certain atypical cases.

These so-called "outlier" cases were specified in the legislation to include cases in which (1) the length of stay exceeded the mean for the DRG by a fixed number of days or a fixed number of standard deviations, whichever was fewer, or (2) the length-of-stay criterion was not exceeded, but the hospital's adjusted costs for the case exceeded a fixed multiple of the DRG rate, or some other fixed dollar amount, whichever was greater (U.S. Congress 1992). This directive to the Secretary of DHHS left considerable flexibility for the department to establish exactly what would constitute either a "day" or a "cost" outlier by how the rules were written. Furthermore, under the terms of the directive, DHHS, as the implementing organization, was left free to modify the definition of an outlier case if it chose to do so—that is, DHHS could change the regulations if it chose to do so.

The regulations promulgated over the years by the DHHS in its implementation of the outlier payment provision of P.L. 98-213 illustrate just how powerful a modifying force rulemaking can be. The chronology of relevant regulations, as cited in the *Federal Register* and subsequently codified in the *Code of Federal Regulations*, includes:

- *49 FR 234.* (Note: The form of these citations is Volume 49, of the *Federal Register*, page 234.) Under this regulation, which applied to fiscal year 1984, the first year of operation for the PPS, the DHHS defined a "day" outlier case as one for which the length of stay exceeded the average length of stay for a particular DRG by the lesser of 20 days or 1.94 standard deviations. It defined a "cost" outlier case to be one in which the hospital's adjusted costs exceeded the greater of 1.5 times the payment amount for the DRG or $12,000.

- *49 FR 3472.* This regulation updated the outlier thresholds for both "day" and "cost" outlier cases and added an element permitting a hospital that transferred a high-cost patient on or after 1 October 1984 to receive "cost" outlier payment.

- *50 FR 35645.* This 1985 regulation updated the outlier thresholds for both "day" and "cost" cases.

- *51 FR 42229.* This regulation was promulgated to implement certain provisions of the Omnibus Budget Reconciliation Act of

1986 (P.L. 99-509) that pertained to payment for outliers. An especially important modification contained in this final rule was the establishment of separate urban and rural outlier payments.

- *53 FR 38476.* This 1988 regulation modified the thresholds used in determining whether a case was a day outlier (24 days or 3 standard deviations above the DRG average) or a cost outlier ($28,000 or 2 times the DRG rate).
- *54 FR 36452.* This regulation, affecting fiscal year 1990, again modified the outlier thresholds. The new threshold for length-of-stay outliers was increased to 28 days or 3 standard deviations; the new threshold for cost outliers became $34,000 or 2 times the DRG rate.
- *55 FR 35990.* The thresholds were again modified for 1991. Length-of-stay outliers were defined as the lesser of 29 days or 3 standard deviations; cost outliers were defined as the greater of $35,000 or 2 times the DRG rate established under the PPS.
- *56 FR 43196.* The thresholds were again increased for 1992: 32 days or 3 standard deviations and $43,000 or 2 times the PPS payment.

This pattern of threshold updates continues and will likely do so in the future unless perhaps it is interrupted by some major modification in the PPS or in other aspects of the Medicare program.

The pattern of using rulemaking to modify policies by updating or changing features of policies, which is exhibited in the regulations used in implementing the PPS policy on payment for outlier cases, is but one example of this very pervasive means of policy modification. Most legislation triggers rulemaking to support its implementation. As was discussed in Chapter 4, rules and regulations promulgated by executive branch agencies and departments to guide policy implementation have the force of law. The rules and regulations themselves are policies. As implementation occurs, the rulemaking mechanism becomes a means to modify policies and their implementation over time. In the process, rulemaking creates new policies. But rulemaking is not the only stage in the implementation phase where modification occurs.

Modification at the policy operation stage

As stated before, policy operation involves the actual running of the programs embedded in enacted legislation. Policy operation is primarily a management process. The managers responsible for policy operation have opportunities to modify policies, especially in terms of their impact, by the manner in which they manage the operation of policies. Policies that are implemented by managers who are committed to the goals of the policies and who have talent and resources available to vigorously implement them are qualitatively different from policies operated by managers who are not committed to the goals of the policies or who lack adequate talent and resources to achieve their full and effective implementation. An example is the best way to illustrate this point.

An example of modification at the policy operation stage

For this example we will use a hypothetical, but plausible scenario of the operation of a policy to immunize the entire American population against AIDS. This hypothetical scenario has been proposed by Levin (1993) as a means to illustrate just how important the policy-operation stage is in policymaking, including the opportunties it provides to modify policies.

Our scenario must, of course, begin with the much-hoped-for day in the future when a fully effective vaccine capable of preventing people from becoming infected with the human immunodeficiency virus (HIV) might be discovered. Following an expedited Food and Drug Administration (FDA) approval (a pattern already established in the late 1980s when pressure from those demanding rapid access to new drugs with potential efficacy in treating AIDS caused the FDA to reconsider its lengthy approval process), our scenario calls for the swift enactment of a federal law setting forth a policy of vaccinating every man, woman, and child in the United States with the new vaccine and the completion of the first round of rulemaking to guide the implementation of such a policy. In our scenario, in other words, we find ourselves at the stage of policy operation where we have the opportunity to consider the potential modifying influence of the manner in which a policy is operationalized on the policy itself.

To some extent our consideration of the policy modification potential inherent in policy operation in this hypothetical scenario about operating a policy of AIDS vaccination can be informed by the real experiences of the 1976 policy to vaccinate the American population against the swine flu virus (Silverstein 1981). However, for the most part, these episodes of policy operation are likely to be quite different and we must rely on our ability to anticipate the problems that are likely to occur in implementing the AIDS vaccination policy as well as how those persons with implementation responsibility might act in the face of these problems. We can, however, be certain that their decisions and actions will be one of the mechanisms through which the policy will be modified for better or worse. A number of problems can be anticipated (Levin 1993).

For example, we can reasonably anticipate that even though the FDA will have approved the vaccine for human use, it might have done so under pressure and without absolute certainty about nor agreement within the scientific community concerning the vaccine's safety and efficacy. This will invite continuing speculation about the vaccine's safety and efficacy. Possible side-effects of the vaccine will be identified and debated in the scientific community; these will probably be substantive debates because such a vaccine is likely to have some potentially serious negative side-effects. Professional judgments will be expressed openly in the media, and because they will not be uniform, many members of the general public will be confused.

We might also anticipate that the focus of media attention will include the scientific controversy over the vaccine's safety and efficacy, and that media attention will probably extend considerably beyond this issue. They will likely scrutinize the controversies that will surely arise over the plans for distributing the vaccine.

For example, an important issue likely to be widely treated in the media would concern the question of who gets the vaccine first. Should it go first to those at highest risk, even if their own behaviors place them at risk? Should the first-available supplies of the vaccine be concentrated in those geographical locations where HIV has had its most devastating impact, even though that is where the heaviest concentrations of already infected people, people for whom a preventative vaccine will offer no protection, are located? Whose ethical or political values will guide such operational decisions?

We can reasonably anticipate that, in the face of uncertainty, the vaccine's manufacturers will demand to be indemnified from suits that will arise from the use or misuse of the vaccine. Perhaps some of those who will administer the vaccine, including private practitioners and public health clinics, will seek protection from legal actions as well. Insurance companies, both those insurers who sell liability protection to the vaccine's manufacturers and distributors and those insurers who may be required under the vaccination policy to pay for the provision of the vaccine to their subscribers, will have strong interests in the policy and preferences for how it is operated. Addressing their interests and preferences will be important components of the operation of this policy.

How such problems as those arising from the scientific controversies over the vaccine's safety and efficacy, the plans for distributing the vaccine, and indemnification for those who manufacture and distribute it are managed will have a great deal to do with the ultimate success or failure of the policy. Those operating the policy will either be able to effectively manage the problems or not. Their degree of success or failure will bear on the policy's impact in a direct way. In addition, their experience with these problems could lead them to modify the regulations governing the policy's implementation and their reporting to legislative bodies with oversight responsibility for this policy could lead to legislative modification of the policy. In these ways the policy itself will be modified.

As we have seen, many, indeed most, health policies in the United States are the result of modification of prior policies. Modification occurs at both the agenda-setting and legislation-development stages of policy formulation and at both the rulemaking and policy operation stages of the implementation phase. The phenomenon of policy modification pervades the entire policymaking process.

Structural Features of the Modification Phase

Much of the activity in the modification phase is driven by two of the phase's structural features. The first of these is the role of oversight actors in the modification process. The second important feature is the role evaluation plays in policy modification.

The role of oversight actors in modification

Oversight actors include the legislative branch, which assigns oversight responsibilities to certain committees and subcommittees, the chief executive (president, governor, or mayor) and the chief executive's top appointees, and the courts. These oversight actors monitor implementation and can serve to point out when adjustments and modifications are needed, or when the results of one policy infringe on or even conflict with the desired results of other policies.

In the case of Congress, and with parallel arrangements in many of the state legislatures, committees and subcommittees have specific oversight responsibilities. The purpose of oversight in this context "is to analyze and evaluate both the execution and effectiveness of laws administered by the executive branch, and to determine if there are areas in which additional legislation (including amendment of existing legislation) is necessary or desirable" (National Health Council, Inc. 1993, 10). While any committee with health jurisdiction can hold oversight hearings, the House and Senate Appropriations Committees have especially important oversight responsibilities inherent in their annual reviews of the budgets of implementing organizations and agencies. Routinely, the budget review mechanism is used by legislators seeking to influence implementation decisions. In addition, out of oversight hearings often come the first or clarifying indications that existing legislation needs to be amended or that new legislation may be needed in a particular area.

The chief executive plays a very important oversight role. In fact, no one else has the power of the chief executive to initiate the modification of policies. In the context of oversight of the implementation of policies, the chief executive role is filled by the president, governor, or mayor but also includes the staff in the Executive Office as well as the appointees in the various departments and agencies who are responsible to the chief executive.

The courts are a third category of oversight actors whose responsibilities include having a role in modifying health policy. The federal courts play an important oversight role regarding how laws are interpreted and enforced. State courts, as well, are involved in interpreting and enforcing state laws and other policies within their jurisdictions. Regarding the role of the federal courts, however, it has been observed

> that a fierce struggle is currently raging over the courts' role in interpreting federal statutes, particularly laws about federal spending for health and other social programs. The intensity of the debate recalls the New Deal constitutional crisis of the 1930s and involves similarly fundamental issues: the norms of legal interpretation, the concept of the judge's role, and the sources and meaning of legal rights. On one side of this debate stands a vision of law that recognizes important rights implicit in the modern welfare state, and sees courts as the legitimate interpreters and enforcers of these rights. These rights include fair agency procedures for deciding individual cases, agency policies that reflect the choices and values embodied in legislation (or, on occasion, the Constitution), and, where appropriate, particular benefits or outcomes. On the other side stands a vision of law that denies the existence of these rights if they are only implicit or based on interpretation, and commands the federal courts to refuse their enforcement unless Congress has defined and required them in super-clear terms. (Rosenblatt 1993, 440)

The existence of a debate over the courts' role implies that their role is neither clear-cut, nor universally agreed on. However, the impact of the courts on the nation's health policy has been significant and will continue to be so. Anderson (1992) has emphasized the courts' recent roles in the modification of health policies in four areas: (1) coverage decisions made by public and private health insurers; (2) states' payment rates for hospitals and nursing homes; (3) antitrust rulings relating to hospital mergers; and (4) the development of criteria to assess the charitable mission of tax-exempt hospitals. These relatively newer areas where the courts have been involved in policy modification are added to the more traditional areas of their involvement. One of the more important of these, for example, is the exercise of their oversight responsibilities in implementing the nation's environmental protection policies. This traditionally important area has been exemplified in the courts' role in implementation of the nation's occupational health and safety laws, which has resulted in numerous modifications of policies in this area.

The Occupational Safety and Health Act (P.L. 91-596) set into motion a massive federal program of standard setting and enforcement that sought to improve safety and health conditions in the nation's workplaces. As Thompson (1981) has noted, "Business and labor leaders . . . have repeatedly appealed decisions by the Occupational Safety and Health Administration (OSHA) to the courts. The development of this program in some respects reads like a legal history" (24). While the courts have their most direct modifying impact on the implementation of policies, especially in ensuring that laws and supporting rules and provisions are appropriately applied, enough adverse judicial decisions growing out of a particular policy can lead to its amendment or even to the stimulation of new legislation.

One of the most troubling aspects of the courts' role in policy modification arises from the fact that the court system in the United States is highly decentralized. Although court autonomy is an important element in the ability of courts to play their roles in the American system of government, one consequence of this autonomy is the possibility of inconsistency in the treatment of policy-relevant issues. As has been noted, "The structure of the judicial system has made it difficult for the courts to provide consistent guidance about what constitutes acceptable behavior" (Anderson 1992, 106).

Limitations of the courts aside, they and the other overseers represent integral structural features of the policymaking process and play important roles in the modification phase of the process.

The role of evaluation in modification

Evaluation is the determination of the worth or value of something—including health policies—judged according to appropriate criteria (House 1993). If the modification of policies is to be most productive, it should be based on solid information including that obtained through evaluation of the policies. Effective policy evaluation, however, is not simply an activity that occurs *after* a policy has been implemented. Policy evaluation is part of a continuum of analytical activities that can begin in the agenda-setting phase and pervade and support the entire policymaking cycle. The continuum of these activities can be organized as ex-ante policy analysis, policy maintenance, policy monitoring, and ex-post policy evaluation (Patton and Sawicki 1993, 369).

Ex-ante policy analysis

This type of analysis, which is also called "anticipatory" or "prospective" policy analysis, occurs mainly in the agenda-setting stage (see

Figure 5.1). This type of analysis helps decision makers to clarify the problems they face, to identify and assess the various potential solutions to the problem, and can include analysis of the relative benefits and costs of the various alternatives for interest groups thereby providing quantitative information that can help decision makers assess the political circumstances of the situation.

Policy maintenance

Sometimes analysis is undertaken to help ensure that policies are implemented as designed and intended. Policy maintenance involves analysis that is part of the exercise of legislative oversight and managerial control. Policy maintenance involves "maintaining the integrity of the policy as it passes out of the (legislative) decision makers' hands into operating agencies or bureaus. The purpose of policy maintenance is not to prevent necessary changes from being made, but to prevent haphazard changes from occurring and to record other purposeful changes in order that they are recognized and can be considered during evaluation" (Patton and Sawicki 1986, 305).

Policy monitoring

This type of analysis is the relatively straightforward measuring and recording of the results of a policy's implementation. As such, policy monitoring takes place within the policy-operation stage of policymaking. However, monitoring is a necessary precursor to the conduct of formal policy evaluations, which help bridge the implementation and modification phases of the policymaking cycle.

Ex-post policy evaluation

Ex-post evaluation, which is also called "retrospective" evaluation, is the process through which the worth or value of a policy is determined. This determination depends on an assessment of the degree to which the objectives established for a policy are achieved through its implementation. Evaluation of policies is a highly technical process that can be approached in a variety of ways. Patton (1981) has identified more than 100 types of evaluation approaches. But generally ex-post policy evaluations are made using one or more of a small number of basic approaches, which includes before-and-after comparisons, with-and-without comparisons, actual-versus-planned performance comparisons, experimental designs, quasi-experimental designs, and cost-oriented policy evaluation approaches. (Patton and Sawicki 1986).

   Before-and-after comparison, as the name suggests, involves comparing conditions or states before a policy is implemented and after it has had an opportunity to make an impact. This is the most widely used approach to policy evaluation.

With-and-without comparison is a modification of the before-and-after approach and involves assessing the conditions in populations or locales with the policy and comparing them to conditions where the policy does not exist. In terms of health policy evaluations, the variation in the states provides a natural laboratory for with-and-without comparisons. For example, a number of studies have been made comparing hospital costs in states with and without rate-setting commissions (Eby and Cohodes 1985).

Actual-versus-planned performance comparison involves comparing post-implementation targets or goals (i.e., dollars saved, people innoculated, tons of solid waste removed, etc.) with actual post-implementation results.

The basic weakness in each of these three types of approaches to ex-post evaluation is that they do not permit the unassailable assignment of causation to the policies being evaluated. They tend to be easy to implement and relatively low-cost evaluation designs, but the results of any of these comparison approaches must be interpreted carefully. To help offset some of the technical limitations and weaknesses of the comparison approaches, two alternative approaches have been developed and are used in some health policy evaluations.

Experimental design usually permits more meaningful comparison. Typically, individuals are randomly assigned to control or experimental groups so that the actual impact of the policy being evaluated can be better assessed: "Although there is and will continue to be a large role for nonexperimental studies, one can clearly have greater confidence in the findings of randomized (experimental) studies" (Newhouse 1991, 191).

One excellent example of the power of experimental designs to evaluate policies can be found in the Health Insurance Experiment conducted by the Rand Corporation in the 1970s (Newhouse 1974). At the time, randomized controlled trials had become the standard approach to clinical research, but the approach had been rarely used in policy evaluation. This important analysis clearly demonstrated the usefulness of the approach for policy evaluation, but the approach is so expensive and difficult to conduct that its impact on policy evaluation remains limited.

Quasi-experimental design is very useful in the world of policy evaluation, especially when a true experiment is too expensive or impractical for other reasons. This approach maintains the logic of full experimentation but without some of its restrictions and expenses. Extensive treatment of this important approach to policy evaluation can be found in Cook and Campbell's classic book, *Quasi-Experimentation: Design and Analysis Issues for Field Settings* (1979). It is important to remember that the most useful policy evaluation is one that can ascribe causality to a policy, although this is extremely difficult to do. Quasi-experimental designs often provide an approach that permits this to occur.

Cost-oriented policy evaluation approaches represent a final type of approach to policy evaluation. These approaches frequently become important in the context of the search for policies that provide value for scarce public dollars. Cost-benefit analysis (CBA) and cost-effectiveness analysis (CEA) are the two most widely used forms of cost-oriented policy evaluation. In CBA, the evaluation is based on the relationship between the benefits and costs of a particular policy and all costs and benefits are expressed in monetary terms. Such analysis helps answer the fundamentally important evaluation question of whether or not the benefits of a policy are at least worth its costs: "The typical result is a measure of 'net benefits,' that is, the difference between the total monetary input costs of an intervention and the consequences of that intervention, also valued in monetary terms" (Elixhauser et al. 1993, JS2).

In CEA, the evaluation is based on the desire to achieve certain policy objectives in the least costly way. This form of analysis compares alternative policies that might be used to achieve the same or very similar objectives. "In CEA, the results are expressed as the net costs required to produce a certain unit of output measured in terms of health, e.g., lives saved, years of life saved, or quality-adjusted life years" (Elixhauser et al. 1993, JS2–JS3). Much of the health-related policy evaluation use of these techniques has centered on analyses related to the variation in utilization rates and the effectiveness of various medical practices and surgical interventions.

Evaluation responsibility in the federal government

The federal government's involvement in evaluation began with the Great Society programs of the mid-1960s. Within the executive branch, the Office of Management and Budget (OMB) centralizes much of the advocacy for policy evaluation. A 1979 circular issued by OMB reflects a high level of commitment to evaluation:

> All agencies of the Executive Branch of the Federal Government will assess the effectiveness of their programs and the efficiency with which they are conducted and seek improvement on a continuing basis so that Federal management will reflect the most progressive practices of both public and business management and result in service to the public. (OMB Circular A-117, quoted in Rist 1990, 73)

Importantly, OMB evaluations are undertaken at the direction of the executive branch of government. Thus the conduct of evaluations, and the use of the results, varies with the preferences of the elected and appointed leaders of the executive branch. For example, the Reagan administration took a number of concrete steps to reduce the number of evaluations conducted, including asking OMB director David Stockman to suspend Circular A-117.

Reflecting in part the tenuousness of the executive branch's commitment to policy evaluation, as well as the legislative branch's need to have independent evaluations to help assess its policies, the Congress created its own evaluation unit in 1980 (House 1993). The General Accounting Office's (GAO) Division of Program Evaluation and Methodology works directly for Congress (Chelimsky 1990). It conducts evaluations, at the request of members of Congress, of several types: ex-ante analysis of potential policies while they are still in the design stage (i.e., work done in the agenda-setting and legislation-development stages); policy maintenance and monitoring; ex-post policy evaluations to establish the effects of policies in order to help guide decisions about their modification; and very importantly, the U.S. General Accounting Office's evaluation unit also critiques the evaluations provided to Congress by others such as the executive branch or interest groups.

Conclusion

The policy modification phase of the public policymaking process involves the feeding back of the outcomes, perceptions, and consequences of existing policies into the other phases of the process. As the feedback loop depicted in Figure 5.1 shows, policy modification occurs in both the agenda setting and legislation development inherent in policy formulation and in the rulemaking and policy operation stages of policy implementation. The modification phase is an extremely important feature of the process through which health policies are made because most American health policies are the result of modification of prior policies.

There are continuous opportunities for the outcomes, perceptions, and consequences resulting from the implementation of policies to influence the formulation of policies, either through influencing agenda setting or through the amendment of prior legislation. And, routinely, the results of policy implementation lead to modifications in both rulemaking and policy operation.

In a very real sense, as was pointed out in the overview of the policymaking process presented in Chapter 2, the modification phase of policymaking exists because perfection cannot be achieved in the other phases and because policies are established and exist in a dynamic world. Suitable policies made today may become inadequate with biological, cultural, demographic, ecological, economic, ethical, psychological, social, and technological changes in the future. Policy modifications—large and small—that occur within the policymaking process emphasize that the separate components of the process are, in reality, highly interactive and interdependent.

Notes

1. Rich histories of the events leading up to the enactment of these amendments have been written by Marmor (1973) and Feder (1977). Such histories document the often rancorous political debates and philosophical differences that led to the 1965 legislation. That history, however, is not repeated here because our interest lies primarily in the pattern of modifications made in the Medicare policy after its enactment as an example of the modification phase of policymaking. Some of the key modifications that have been made in the Medicare policy since its enactment in 1965 are chronicled in this section.
2. Resource-based relative value scale (RBRVS) is a method of determining physicians' fees based on the time spent in providing services, the skills and training necessary to provide the services, and other factors. The methodology was developed by Harvard economist, William C. Hsiao. See his *A National Study of Resource-Based Relative Values for Physician Services: Final Report*, Washington, DC: Health Care Financing Administration Contract No. 17-C-98795-03, 27 September 1988.

References

Altmeyer, A. J. *The Formative Years of Social Security*. Madison: University of Wisconsin Press, 1968.
Anderson, G. F. "The Courts and Health Policy: Strengths and Limitations." *Health Affairs* 11, no. 4 (Winter 1992): 95–110.
Chelimsky, E. "Expanding GAO's Capabilities in Program Evaluation." *The GAO Journal* (Winter–Spring 1990): 43–52.
Cook, T. P., and D. T. Campbell. *Quasi-Experimentation: Design and Analysis Issues for Field Settings*. Chicago: Rand McNally, 1979.
Eby, C. L., and D. R. Cohodes. "What Do We Know About Rate-Setting?" *Journal of Health Politics, Policy and Law* 10, no. 2 (Summer 1985): 299–327.
Elixhauser, A., B. R. Luce, W. R. Taylor, and J. Reblando. "Health Care CBA/CEA: An Update on the Growth and Composition of the Literature." *Medical Care* 31, no. 7 (Supplement 1993): JS1–11.
Feder, J. *Medicare: The Politics of Federal Hospital Insurance*. Lexington, MA: Lexington Books, 1977.
House, E. R. *Professional Evaluation: Social Impact and Political Consequences*. Newbury Park, CA: Sage Publications, 1993.
Levin, M. A. "The Day After an AIDS Vaccine is Discovered: Management Matters." *Journal of Policy Analysis and Management* 12, no. 3 (Summer 1993): 438–55.
Lindblom, C. E. "The Science of Muddling Through." *Public Administration Review* 14 (Spring 1959): 79–88.

Marmor, T. R. *The Politics of Medicare*. Chicago: Aldine, 1973.

National Health Council, Inc. *Congress and Health: An Introduction to the Legislative Process and Its Key Participants*, 10th ed. Government Relations Handbook Series. New York: National Health Council, Inc., 1993.

Newhouse, J. P. "Controlled Experimentation as Research Policy." In *Health Services Research: Key to Health Policy*, edited by E. Ginzberg, 161–94. Cambridge, MA: Harvard University Press, 1991.

————. "A Design for a Health Insurance Experiment" *Inquiry* 11, no. 1 (1974): 5–27.

Patton, C. V., and D. Sawicki. *Basic Methods of Policy Analysis and Planning*, 2d ed.. Englewood Cliffs, NJ: Prentice-Hall, 1993.

Patton, M. Q. *Creative Evaluation*. Beverly Hills, CA: Sage Publications, 1981.

Peterson, M. A. "Political Influence in the 1990s: From Iron Triangles to Policy Networks." *Journal of Health Politics, Policy and Law* 18, no. 2 (Summer 1993): 395–438.

Rhodes, R. P. *Health Care Politics, Policy, and Distributive Justice*. Albany: State University of New York Press, 1992.

Rist, R. C., editor. *Program Evaluation and the Management of Government*. New Brunswick, NJ: Transaction Books, 1990.

Rosenblatt, R. E. "The Courts, Health Care Reform, and the Reconstruction of American Social Legislation." *Journal of Health Politics, Policy and Law* 18, no. 2 (Summer 1993): 439–76.

Russell, L. B., and C. L. Manning. "The Effect of Prospective Payment on Medicare Expenditures." *New England Journal of Medicine* 320, no. 7 (16 February 1989): 439–44.

Silverstein, A. M. *Pure Politics and Impure Science*. Baltimore: The Johns Hopkins University Press, 1981.

Starr, P. *The Social Transformation of American Medicine*. New York: Basic Books, 1982.

Starr, P., and W. A. Zelman. "Bridge to Compromise: Competition Under a Budget." *Health Affairs* 12 (Supplement 1993): 7–23.

Thompson, F. J. *Health Policy and the Bureaucracy: Politics and Implementation*. Cambridge: The Massachusetts Institute of Technology Press, 1981.

U.S. Congress. House Committee on Ways and Means. *1992 Green Book*. Washington, DC: U.S. Government Printing Office, 1992.

6

The Other Side of Policymaking

$\mathbf{A}$s the model of the health policymaking process used throughout this book illustrates (see Figures 2.1, 3.1, 4.1, and 5.1), the process yields outcomes, perceptions, and consequences. But, for whom? Thus far, the important question of who feels the end-results of the policymaking process has only been discussed indirectly. To fully understand this process, however, it is necessary to consider who the process affects, as well as the implications for them and for the process itself.

The obvious answer to the question of who is affected by the health policymaking process is, of course, everyone. People affected by the process share, to varying degrees, two related concerns about it: First, they want to know how policies will impact on them and on the people and things that they care about or for which they are responsible. In other words, people have a discernment concern. People normally want information about anything that affects them, including health policies—and they prefer this information in advance of the impact. Second, they want to have some ability to influence the policies that impact on them. These impacts can, after all, be quite direct and of real consequence. As a result of specific policies, for instance, certain people gain or lose access to a particular medical procedure, obtain or fail to obtain grants to support research projects, see their incomes rise or fall, or see their taxes increased.

The ability to discern the impact of policies, especially if it is to be done in advance and with specificity, can almost always be increased through the pooling of resources. This is true whether the people involved are individual health professionals, managers responsibile for health care organizations, technology producers, individual consumers, or taxpayers. Even more so, the ability of individuals to influence the policies that impact on them can be greatly enhanced through collective action. Thus, it is no accident that most efforts intended to discern the potential impact of policies as well as those efforts intended to influence the policymaking process are made through organizations. And, as we will see, such efforts are made through many different types of organizations.

The fact that organizations play such vital roles in discerning the impact of policies and in influencing them, is not to say that individuals, as individuals, have no means to discern impact or influence policies. People can and do follow the policymaking process closely through the news media and perhaps through personal contact. And they can and do exert influence on policymaking by their votes, their financial contributions to the campaigns of favored candidates for political office, and by the policymakers and causes they work for and support. But there is no question that discernment and influence are both enhanced by resources that only organizations, which are after all only collections of individuals, can bring to bear on these tasks.

The relationship between health policies and the organizations on which they impact is quite direct. The clearest way to visualize this relationship is to recognize that the ultimate performance outcomes achieved by organizations—whether measured in terms of financial strength, reputation, growth, competititve position, services provided, or some other parameter—begin with and are heavily influenced by the nature of the opportunties and threats imposed on organizations from their external environments. This relationship is depicted in Figure 6.1.

The external environments faced by organizations include biological, cultural, demographic, ecological, economic, ethical, legal, political, psychological, social, and technological dimensions. Policies that affect an organization are only part of its external environment, but they constitute a critically important part. As Figure 6.1 illustrates, policies, along with the other variables in an organization's external environment, provide the organization with a set of opportunities and threats to which it can—indeed, must—respond.

The organization responds to the threats and opportunities presented to it by its external environment with strategies and with organizational structures created to carry out the strategies. Strategies and structures result in organizational performance. But the series of events that culminates in organizational performance is triggered by the opportunties and threats the organization faces. And these opportunities and threats are the direct result of conditions in the organization's external environment, including the policies that impact on the organization.

Given the importance of their external environments, including policies, to their ultimate performance, organizations on which health policies impact usually develop strong operational commitments both to discerning policies' impacts and to influencing them. They pursue these commitments by developing information about policies in advance of

Figure 6.1 The Relationship between an Organization's External
Environment and Its Performance

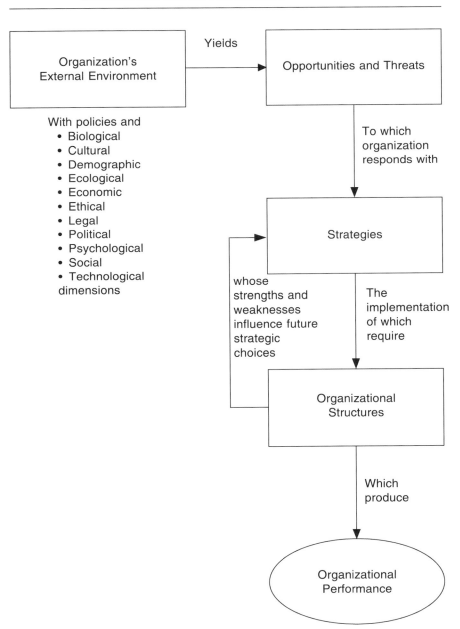

their impact so that preparations and adjustments can be made and by seeking to influence the formulation, implementation, and modification of relevant policies.

This chapter explores the two principal concerns that organizations and the people who populate them have about health policies—discernment and influence—and considers the actions they take as a result of these concerns. First, however, it will be useful to consider the variety of these organizations and the specific nature of their health policy concerns in a systematic way.

Organizations Affected by Health Policies

A rich variety of organizations populates the health policy community. All of these organizations are affected by and have concerns about health policies. The diversity of these organizations defies easy categorization, although the most obvious category includes organizations that provide health services. Hospitals, state or county health departments, HMOs, hospices, and nursing homes are examples. This category can be called primary provider organizations.

Another category consists of secondary provider organizations. These are organizations that produce resources for the primary providers to use in the conduct of their work. Examples of secondary providers are educational institutions that help produce the health care system's workforce, organizations such as Blue Cross plans and commercial insurance firms that facilitate payment for health care services, and pharmaceutical and medical supply companies among many others.

Another category of organizations with health policy concerns are the associations and professional societies that represent the primary and secondary providers. These organizations, whose memberships are comprised of individual professionals (e.g., the American Medical Association (AMA) or the American Association for Respiratory Care) or comprised of organizations (e.g., the American Hospital Association (AHA) or the Pharmaceutical Research and Manufacturers of America (PhRMA)), represent the interests of their members.

A final category of organizations with health policy concerns are consumer groups. Consumers have concerns about the impact of health policies on their health as well as on their finances. Employers, who provide health insurance benefits, share these concerns of their employees. In fact, given the extent to which employers provide health insurance benefits, many consumer concerns about health policies are addressed through employers or through associations such as the Chamber of Business and Industry that represent employers. In addition, however, a wide variety of consumer groups such as the American Association of Retired Persons (AARP), Citizen Action, the National Council of Senior Citizens, Families U.S.A., or the Consortium for Citizens With Disabilities also represent certain categories of consumers.

In the following sections, these different categories of organizations will be briefly described and their health policy concerns outlined. The final sections of the chapter will explore the actions these organizations take in pursuit of their dual concerns about discerning the impact of policies and influencing policies.

Organizations that provide health care services (primary providers)

Organizations in this category share the distinguishing characteristic of providing the structures within which the delivery of health care services is made directly to consumers, whether the purpose of the services is preventive, curative, restorative, or continuing care.

One way to visualize the diversity of primary providers is to consider a comprehensive continuum of clinical health care services, a continuum extending from before birth to after death. Adapting a chronological list developed by Cummings and Abell (1993), the list of such services includes:

- Organizations and programs that seek to minimize negative environmental impact on health
- Family planning services
- Prenatal counseling services
- Prenatal ambulatory care facilities
- Birthing facilities
- Well-baby nurseries contiguous with the birthing facilities and centralized neonatal intensive care units (NICUs) in affilitated hospitals
- Pediatric outpatient clinic services
- Pediatric inpatient hospital facilities, including NICUs and pediatric ICUs (intensive care units)
- Child and adolescent psychiatric inpatient and outpatient facilities
- Adult outpatient facilities
- Adult inpatient hospital facilities, including cardiac care units, surgical intensive care units, monitored units, "transition" beds, and emergency departments

- Cancer units (stand-alone with radiotherapy capability and short-stay recovery beds)
- Rehabilitation inpatient and outpatient facilities, including specific subprograms for orthopedic, neurological, cardiac, arthritis, speech, otologic, and other services
- Psychiatric inpatient and outpatient facilities, including specific subprograms for psychotics, day programs, counseling services (adult and adolescent), and detoxification
- Home health care facilities and programs, including specific subprograms for newborns, children, and adults
- Skilled and intermediate nursing facilities
- Adult day care facilities
- Respite facilities for caregivers of homebound pediatric and adult patients, including services such as the provision of meals, visiting nurse and home health aides, electronic emergency call capability, cleaning, and simple home maintenance
- Hospice care facilities and associated family services, including bereavement, legal, and financial counseling.

The continuum of health care services outlined above has traditionally been provided almost exclusively by autonomous organizations. And the services have often been provided in an uncoordinated and disjointed way. However, the health care system is undergoing a revolution in terms of how the primary provider organizations are related to each other. Vertical integration, in which many of the facilities listed above are joined together into unified organizational arrangments, is reshaping the nation's system of primary provider organizations (Mick and Conrad 1988). This phenomenon can be expected to intensify under the impetus of the health reforms initiated in the early 1990s.

Voluntary accrediting organizations

An important subset of organizations in this cateogory exists because many types of primary provider organizations seek voluntary accreditation as a means of improving themselves and of ensuring the public of their adherence to a set of rigorous standards. These accrediting organizations also have interests in health policy.

Among a number of organizations that accredit primary providers, none is more important than the Joint Commission on Accreditation of Healthcare Organizations (JCAHO). The Joint Commission can trace its origin to a 1918 program of the American College of Surgeons (ACS) through which that organization surveyed hospitals in the United States for the purpose of upgrading the quality of medical care provided in them. In 1951, the ACS was joined by several other organizations, such as the AHA and the AMA in forming the Joint Commission. Using standards established by professional and technical advisory committees, the JCAHO accredits health care services provider organizations that voluntarily seek such accreditation and thus guides and influences much of the operation of these organizations.

The Joint Commission lists several benefits of accreditation for a primary provider organization:

- Identification of strengths and weaknesses with particular attention to areas in which performance may be improved
- On-site education and consultation
- Increased staff morale and enhanced ability to recruit professional staff
- Public recognition of the organization's commitment to quality
- Eligibility for reimbursement by many third-party payers
- Immediate eligibility to participate in the Medicare program
- Recognition, in most states, of compliance with state licensure requirements. (Joint Commission on Accreditation of Healthcare Organizations 1990, 10)

The policy concerns of primary provider organizations

The generic concerns of organizations that provide health services involve the discernment of policy changes and developments that might affect the organizations, as well as the desire to exert influence over the policies affecting them. The attention of primary provider organizations, however, tends to be sharply focused on policies that directly affect their prospects, decisions, and actions in a number of specific areas. Key among these are issues of access to and cost of health services. But other important areas include financing and reimbursement arrangements; the structure of the delivery system, including antitrust issues involved in mergers and consolidations; meeting the needs of special populations; assuring quality; and a number of ethical and legal issues that arise in providing access to affordable health services of an appropriate quality to all who need them (Crane, Hersh, and Shortell 1992).

In addition to these areas of explicit concern, primary provider organizations are also generally concerned about the policy issues that affect the organizations that produce resources for them or that represent them, as well as about individual consumers and groups of consumers— people who are, after all, their customers.

Organizations that produce resources
for health care (secondary providers)

The organizations in this category produce and distribute resources that are used by the primary providers in providing health care services. These secondary providers include educational institutions and programs, insurance organizations that provide reimbursement services for providers as well as insurance protection for consumers, and the pharmaceutical and medical supply companies.

Educational institutions

A wide variety of educational organizations and programs supply human resources who are employed in the pursuit of health. As was noted in Chapter 1, approximately 10.6 million people work in the health sector. Many of them are prepared in specialized educational institutions and programs. Medical schools and nursing schools are prominent examples, although many other educational institutions contribute vital human resources.

The majority of the nation's physicians are educated in its 126 allopathic and 15 osteopathic medical schools. But foreign medical graduates (FMGs) educated in other countries continue to be an important source of physicians for the United States. Approximately 130,000, or about 22 percent of the 600,000 licensed physicians in the country at present are FMGs (Mick and Moscovice 1993).

The basic model of physician education is a four-year postbaccalaureate program leading to the M.D. or D.O. degree, followed by several years of postgraduate training in a residency. The residency years are called postgraduate years and are numbered sequentially as PG-I, PG-II, etc. These years are spent in teaching hospitals. The medical specialties determine the number of postgraduate years and the specific clinical content of those years as the basis for certification in that specialty. For example, anesthesiology requires that PG-I be spent in a general residency and PG-II through PG-IV be spent in an anesthesiology residency program. The family practice specialty requires three years to be spent in a family practice residency; neurological surgery requires one year of general residency and five years of neurological surgery residency. Residency programs are accredited by the Accreditation Council for Graduate Medical Education (ACGME), which is composed of professional medical associations. Each specialty sets standards for its specialty training through its residency review committee. Both medical schools and teaching hospitals have health policy interests.

The nation's registered nurses (RNs) are educated in 489 baccalaureate programs, 829 associate degree programs, and 152 hospital-based diploma programs (National League for Nursing 1991). Following completion of one of these approved programs, a nurse can become a registered nurse by passing a state licensure examination. Every state and the District of Columbia have mandatory licensing statutes.

There are also masters- and doctoral-level education programs for nurses, providing them with advanced training in education, research, and administration, or in such clinical nursing specialties as public health, medical-surgical nursing, mental health, maternal and child health, and cardiovascular nursing. Other specialty training includes programs for nurse anesthetists, nurse-midwives, and pediatric and family nurse practitioners. A pediatric nurse practitioner, for example, is a registered nurse who has received additional training permitting an expanded role in the care of pediatric patients. Many nurses with advanced training are finding new roles in HMOs, ambulatory surgery centers, and home care programs providing care for elderly patients and patients with chronic illnesses. RNs are also increasingly involved in utilization management and quality review roles in health care organizations. The organizations that educate and employ nurses have interests in policies that affect the supply of nurses.

Voluntary Educational Accreditation Agencies. A subset of this category of secondary provider organizations includes organizations that accredit the educational institutions and programs that supply human resources to the health care system. Educational accreditation is a process whereby a private, nongovernmental organization reviews an educational institution or a specialized school or program of study against a set of established qualifications and standards.

Graduate programs for the education of managers for the health care system can voluntarily seek accreditation by the Accrediting Commission on Education for Health Services Administration (ACEHSA). The board of ACEHSA includes representatives from the American College of Healthcare Executives (ACHE), the AHA, the Association of University Programs in Health Administration (AUPHA), the American College of Health Care Administrators, the American College of Medical Group Administrators, the Association of Mental Health Administrators, the American Public Health Association, and a joint seat occupied by the Canadian Hospital Association and the Canadian College of Health Service Executives.

The National League for Nursing (NLN) accredits schools of nursing, the Commission on Accreditation of the American Dental Association accredits dental schools, and medical education at different levels (M.D. programs, graduate medical education, and continuing medical education) is subject to accreditation by organizations including the American Board of Medical Specialties, AMA, Association for Hospital

Medical Education, Association of American Medical Colleges, and the Council of Medical Specialty Societies. These and other organizations involved in educational accreditation have health policy interests.

The policy concerns of educational institutions and accreditors

These organizations are concerned with policies that affect the resources used in educating health professionals, in licensure and practice guideline policies, and indirectly, in policies that affect the demand for their graduates. But beyond these obvious and long-standing policy concerns, are some newer and less obvious concerns. Given the crucial role health care practitioners play in the nation's health, increasing attention is being given to the competencies these people should possess if they are to make their maximum contributions to health. One such analysis has been made by the Pew Health Professions Commission, a privately supported effort involving leaders from many of the health professions. According to this commission (Shugars, O'Neil, and Bader 1991), future health care practitioners should

- *Care for the community's health*—Practitioners should have a broad understanding of the determinants of health such as environment, socioeconomic conditions, behavior, medical care and genetics and be able to work with others in the community to integrate a range of services and activities that promote, protect, and improve health.
- *Expand access to effective care*—Practitioners should participate in efforts to ensure access to health care for individuals, families, and communities and to improve the public's health.
- *Provide contemporary clinical care*—Practitioners should possess up-to-date clinical skills to meet the public's health care needs.
- *Emphasize primary care*—Practitioners should be willing and able to function in new health care settings and interdisciplinary team arrangements designed to meet the primary health care needs of the public.
- *Participate in coordinated care*—Practitioners should be able to work effectively as team members in organized settings that emphasize high-quality, cost-effective integrated services.
- *Ensure cost-effective and appropriate care*—Practitioners should incorporate and balance cost and quality in the decision-making process.
- *Practice prevention*—Practitioners should emphasize primary and secondary preventive strategies for all people. ["*Primary* prevention involves prevention of the disease or injury itself. Improved highway design, school education programs concerning smoking and substance abuse, and immunization against poliomyelitis or measles are examples of primary prevention. *Secondary* prevention blocks progression of an injury or disease from an impairment to a disability. Use of the Papanicolaou smear to look for early cellular changes that are thought

to be precursors of cancer is a good example of secondary prevention. An impairment has already occurred, but disability may be prevented through early intervention" (Pickett and Hanlon 1990, 83)].

- *Involve patients and families in the decision-making process*—Practitioners should expect patients and their families to participate actively both in decisions regarding their personal health care and in evaluating its quality and acceptability.

- *Promote healthy lifestyles*—Practitioners should help individuals, families and communities maintain and promote healthy behavior.

- *Assess and use technology appropriately*—Practitioners should understand and apply increasingly complex and often costly technology and use it appropriately.

- *Improve the health care system*—Practitioners should understand the determinants and operations of the health system from a broad political, economic, social and legal [and ethical] perspective in order to continuously improve the operations and accountability of that system.

- *Manage information*—Practitioners should manage and use large volumes of scientific, technological and patient information.

- *Understand the role of the physical environment*—Practitioners should be prepared to assess, prevent and mitigate the impact of environmental hazards on the health of the population.

- *Provide counseling on ethical issues*—Practitioners should provide counseling for patients in situations where ethical issues arise, as well as participate in discussions of ethical issues in health care as they affect communities, society and the health professions.

- *Accommodate expanded accountability*—Practitioners should be responsive to increasing levels of public, governmental and third party participation in and scrutiny of the shape and direction of the health care system.

- *Participate in a racially and culturally diverse society*—Practitioners should appreciate the growing diversity of the population and the need to understand health status and health care through differing cultural values.

- *Continue to learn*—Practitioners should anticipate changes in health care and respond by redefining and maintaining professional competency throughout practice life. (18–20) (Reprinted with permission as it appeared in Shugars, D. A., O'Neil, E. H., and Bader, J. D., eds. *Healthy America: Practitioners for 2005, An Agenda for Action for U.S. Health Professional Schools.* Durham, NC: The Pew Health Professions Commission © 1991.)

The education and deployment of health care practitioners who possess these competencies will be affected not only by policies that affect a broad range of issues related specifically to the education of these practitioners, but also by policies that relate more generally to the costs of operating the health care system, providing access to its services, and assuring the quality of those services. The secondary providers obviously share these concerns with the primary providers.

Organizations that provide health insurance

A second important category of organizations that provide resources for the nation's pursuit of health are those whose services facilitate payment for care. There are three types of health insurance in the United States: (1) voluntary, private health insurance, which is provided through either Blue Cross and Blue Shield plans, commercial insurance companies, or HMOs; (2) social health insurance, which is one of several types of government entitlement programs, usually linked to previous employment—worker's compensation insurance and the Medicare program are examples of social health insurance; and (3) public welfare, of which the Medicaid program is the most important example (Koch 1993).

Approximately 86 percent of the population of the United States has some form of health insurance coverage. About 74 percent of the population is covered by private health insurance (61 percent through employers and 13 percent by the direct purchase of nongroup insurance). Approximately 13 percent of the population has coverage through the Medicare program, 10 percent through the Medicaid program and 4 percent through the military or veterans' program. Fourteen percent of the population is uninsured. It should be noted that these percentages total more than 100 percent because some people have more than one type of health insurance coverage (De Lew, Greenberg, and Kinchen 1992).

More than 1,000 private health insurance companies provide health insurance policies of several types, including: hospital/medical insurance, major medical expense insurance, Medicare supplemental insurance, disability income protection, dental expense insurance, and long-term care insurance. Prepaid health plans, HMOs in particular, are a rapidly growing segment of the private health insurance market in the United States. There are approximately 600 HMOs in the country today, enrolling more than 33 million people.

Private health insurance companies are regulated by the states through insurance commissioners. State policies regarding reserves to be held by insurance companies, mandated benefit structures, premiums, and rules for paying the insured or health care services providers can vary considerably from one state to another. Employer-provided health insurance coverage has been encouraged by federal tax policy. Contributions paid by employers for health insurance for their employees and their dependents are basically a substitute for cash wages. But these payments are not subject to personal income tax nor to the Social Security tax. If these contributions had been taxed as income in 1990, it would have generated approximately $56 billion in Federal revenues (Employee Benefit Research Institute 1991).

The policy concerns of health insurers

One of the recurrent policy concerns of private health insurance organizations involves maintaining the antitrust immunity they received under the 1945 federal McCarran-Ferguson Act (P.L. 79-15). They are also obviously concerned about their future role in any federally driven reform of the nation's health care system. But because health insurers are regulated at the state level, much of their policy interest is focused at this level. The Health Insurance Association of America (1990), an association representing commercial health insurance companies, has identified a number of specific policy interests and positions of its members, including:

- Opposing policies mandating that particular medical services be covered by insurance
- Opposing policies restricting the use of consumer cost-sharing
- Supporting policies assuring insurers reasonable access to medical records needed in utilization review activities
- Encouraging Congress to consider policies to reduce subsidies which support capital expansion in the health system through prohibiting tax exemption of interest earned on bonds used to finance construction and equipment in the system
- Supporting policies through which government provides data to consumers, payers, and purchasers of health care services to help in their assessments of health outcomes and the cost and quality of care
- Supporting policies limiting the supply of physicians and bringing the specialty distribution of physicians more into line with the health needs of the population
- Supporting policies reducing costs associated with malpractice.

Pharmaceutical and medical supply companies

A third category of resource-producing organizations are those found in the pharmaceutical and medical supply industries. National expenditures on the products of these organizations in 1995 will total approximately $100 billion and could reach $150 billion by 2000 (Burner, Waldo, and McKusick 1992). Pharmaceutical companies such as Glaxo, Eli Lilly, Merck, Pfizer, and Schering-Plough have been remarkably profitable enterprises in the United States, and they have made significant contributions to the quest for health. According to the Pharmaceutical Research and Manufacturers of America, there are now more than 30 anti-cancer drugs available in the United States and another 100 drugs are under development to help treat and manage cancer.

The companies that manufacture and distribute medical supplies are as diverse as their products, which range from cotton balls to the most sophisticated imaging equipment. Firms such as Johnson and Johnson, Baxter International, Abbott Labs, and Bausch and Lomb make up this industry. In 1993, the nation's three fastest growing industries were x-ray appliances and tubes, electromedical equipment, and surgical-medical instruments (U.S. Department of Commerce 1993). Indeed, technological advances, including medical technology, have long been seen as vital both to the nation's economic growth and to its place on the world's economic stage by business leaders and public officials alike. And technology's economic benefits do not accrue solely to those who produce the technology. Those primary provider organizations, and the individuals within them, using technology in their work also reap direct economic benefits.

The policy concerns of pharmaceutical and medical supply companies

As was discussed in Chapter 3, medical technology, including the products of the pharmaceutical and medical supply industries, is affected by a vast array of policies (review Table 3.1 for examples of such policies). Current policies are driven mainly by three factors. First, medical technology plays an important role in rising health costs. Second, medical technology frequently provides health benefits to people, although it does not always do so. Third, the utilization of medical technology provides economic benefits to certain people quite aside from its potential to provide health benefits. These three factors are likely to remain important determinants of the nation's policies toward medical technology.

While increasing health costs are the result of a variety of variables, technology certainly plays a part. Its role is affected by two interrelated market failures affecting both the production and consumption of medical technology. One failure is the lack of availability of adequate information on technology's costs and benefits. The other is the existence of perverse economic incentives that affect the production and consumption of medical technology, leading to widespread overutilization of this technology. Primarily, these incentives spring from the fee-for-service system of payment, in which provider earnings are directly linked to the volume and type of services provided. High-tech services are generally more lucrative than alternatives. This circumstance is exacerbated by the fact that most patients are insured, so they rarely feel restrained from using recommended technology by economic considerations. In addition, providers' real and perceived concerns about medical liability stimulate the further use of medical technology (U.S. Congressional Budget Office 1991; Durenberger and Foote 1993).

Because of its role in rising health costs, and especially in response to the market failures associated with medical technology, some current policies explicitly seek to address these problems. For example, the Food and Drug Administration is charged to ensure that new pharmaceuticals meet safety and efficacy standards; the peer review organizations (PROs) are intended to ensure that only needed and appropriate procedures are performed on Medicare beneficiaries; and government is spending an increasing amount of money on the conduct of outcome studies that are intended to identify the relative values among alternative technologies, presumably so that it can support the best values in technology.

Each of these examples of current policies, and many others, represent policy responses to the fact that medical technology adds to the expense of health care and that the markets for this technology do not work very well. These types of policies attempt to provide a check or at least some level of inhibition against the unfettered development, diffusion, and use of medical technology, which the marketplace has not adequately provided.

Although the use of medical technology can be costly, its use can also produce health benefits for people. In view of its potential health benefits, a second factor driving the nation's current medical technology policy is a desire on the part of policymakers to foster and facilitate the development and diffusion of beneficial technology and to expand access to it. Thus, we have policies that provide financial support for research and development that might lead to new medical technology and policies such as the Medicare and Medicaid programs to help provide wider access to the technology.

The third factor driving current policy is medical technology's economic role. Medical technology generates costs for consumers, for whom it may or may not produce health benefits. But quite aside from this, medical technology also generates enormous *economic* benefits. These benefits are in the form of revenues for technology producers and for those who use the technology in their work and in the form of taxes on these revenues that are paid to government. Because of its economic role, some policies are intended to make the markets for medical technology work well and fairly. Some of these policies take the form of laws and judicial decisions governing contracts intended to ensure that the economic exchanges that occur within these markets follow predictable patterns. Others take the form of tax laws intended to spur economic activity. Still other policies define and are used to punish antitrust violations.

Clearly, the pharmaceutical and medical supply organizations have wide-ranging health policy interests. Like the primary provider organizations and the other secondary provider organizations discussed earlier, their health policy concerns include discerning changes in these policy areas and exerting their influence on the formulation, implementation, and modification of policies that might have an impact on them.

Organizations that represent primary and secondary providers

As was noted in Chapter 2, one of the most significant features of the political economy of the United States in regard to health policy is the fact that the interests of both primary and secondary provider organizations are highly concentrated. This phenomenon results in the formation of organizations, usually called associations, whose purpose is to serve the collective interests of the members. Such organizations, whose members also usually constitute an interest group, seek to discern policy changes that might affect their members and inform them about such changes. They also seek to influence the formulation, implementation, and modification of policies for the purpose of providing the group's members some advantage. The health policy interests of the associations are defined by the interests of their constituent members.

Primary provider associations

The organizations that provide health care services, such as hospitals and nursing homes, are widely represented by associations. Hospitals can belong to the American Hospital Association (AHA). The AHA was established in 1898 and seeks to represent the interests of its member organizations in the nation's political processes. Reflecting the diversity of the hospital industry, there are associations that represent subsets of hospitals. Examples include the Federation of American Health Systems, whose members are investor-owned hospitals. The Federation's central purpose is to serve as its members' advocate to Congress, the executive branch, the media, academia, and the public. It also serves as the clearinghouse of information from which members and others can obtain information on health matters and industry positions, policies, and statistics. The Catholic Health Association and the Protestant Hospital Association represent subsets of hospitals with sectarian ownership and interests. The Council of Teaching Hospitals and the National Association of Children's Hospitals and Related Institutions represent member institutions with specialized purposes and interests.

The American Health Care Association, established in 1949, is the largest association for long-term care providers in the United States. The Group Health Association of America (GHAA) is the association for all types of HMOs and the Medical Group Management Association (MGMA) represents many of the nation's medical group practices.

In addition to the associations representing primary provider organizations, there are other associations whose membership is comprised of individual practitioners. These associations also seek to serve the individual and collective interests of their members. Physicians can join the American Medical Association (AMA); African-American physicians may choose to join the National Medical Association; women physicians can join the American Medical Women's Association. Physicians also have the opportunity to affiliate with associations, usually termed "colleges" or "academies," where membership is based on medical specialty. Prominent examples are the American College of Surgeons and the American Academy of Pediatrics. Other personal membership associations include the American College of Healthcare Executives, American Nurses Association, American Dental Association, American Podiatry Association, American Psychologcial Association, Association of Operating Room Nurses, National Association of Social Workers, American Pharmaceutical Association, and the American Academy of Physician Assistants.

Often, in addition to national associations, primary provider organizations and individual practitioners can join state and local associations that also represent their interests. For example, every state has a state hospital association and a state medical society. Urban centers and densely populated areas often have associations at the regional or county and sometimes even the city levels. The existence of the hundreds of associations for primary provider organizations and for the practitioners who work within them in the United States are a reflection of the specialization and fragmentation that exist within the health context (Rakich, Longest, and Darr 1992).

Secondary provider associations

In addition to the associations representing primary provider organizations and individual practitioners, the secondary provider organizations also have their own associations. Examples include the Association of American Medical Colleges, Association of University Programs in Health Administration, Blue Cross and Blue Shield Association, Health Insurance Association of America, Pharmaceutical Research and Manufacturers of America, and the Industrial Biotechnology Association, among many others. Like their counterpart associations that represent primary providers, these associations focus on policies that affect their members.

Consumer groups and employers

Reflecting the diversity of the population from which their members are drawn, consumer groups with health care interests are quite varied. Some consumer-oriented associations reflect specific diseases such as the American Cancer Society or the American Heart Association. Others, such as Citizen Action, Families U.S.A., and the Consortium for Citizens With Disabilities, seek to represent the interests of broader groups of people.

The policy concerns of consumer groups and employers

The health policy concerns of consumers and the groups that represent them reflect the rich diversity of the American people. As was noted in Chapter 1, two demographic variables in particular are helping to shape consumers' health needs and thus heavily influence society's views on health policy. These variables are the age structure of the population and its racial and ethnic diversity.

As people age, they consume relatively more health care services and their health care needs differ from those of younger people (Burner, Waldo, and McKusick 1992). They also become more likely to consume long-term care services and community-based services intended to help them cope with various limitations in the activities of daily living. In addition to their unique health needs, older citizens of the United States have a special health policy history and therefore a unique set of expectations and preferences regarding the nation's health policy. The Medicare program described earlier, which includes extensive provisions for health benefits in the context of the nation's social insurance support for its older citizens, is a key feature of this history.

Building on the concentrated interests of older people and their preferences to preserve and extend their health care benefits through public policies, organizations such as the American Association of Retired Persons (AARP) and the National Council of Senior Citizens have become important organizations seeking to serve the health policy interests of their members.

African-Americans and, more recently, the rapidly growing number of Hispanic-Americans, face special health problems. Both groups are underserved for many health care services and under-represented in all of the health professions in the United States. Their health policy interests encompass getting their unique health problems—such as higher infant mortality, higher exposure to violence among adolescents, higher levels of substance abuse among adults, and compared to other segments of the population, earlier deaths from cardiovascular disease and many other causes—adequately addressed.

The health policy concerns of American employers have intensified dramatically in recent years, although their interests are by no means uniform across all employers. To a large extent, their concerns are shaped by the degree to which employers are involved in the provision of health insurance benefits to their employees and their dependents and, in some cases, to large numbers of retirees. Many employers began providing health insurance benefits during World War II when wages were frozen and labor exacted health insurance and other benefits in lieu of wages. Many employers provided insurance benefits that obligated them to cover most of their employees' medical costs—no matter what these costs eventually turned out to be (Longest and Detre 1991).

The cost of providing health insurance coverage is blamed in part for the deteriorating international competitiveness of American business, although opinions about the role of insurance benefit costs in this matter are mixed (U.S. Congressional Budget Office 1992). Whether these costs are to blame or not, employers have clear-cut interests in holding down their operating costs, including those associated with providing health insurance benefits. Thus, any health policies that affect the costs incurred by employers will capture their attention.

But costs are not the only things that drive employers' concerns about health policy. Health insurance benefits are provided to help employers attract and maintain productive workforces. This means that employers are interested in improving the health of their employees. It also means they are interested in preventing work disruptions such as those caused by labor unrest. Thus, health policies that affect the health of workers or the health of the labor-management relations experienced by employers also attract their attention.

Now that the types of organizations with health policy interests have been identified and the areas of policy where their interests are concentrated have been described, we can explore the mechanisms these organizations use to discern policy changes that might impact on them or to influence the policymaking process.

Discerning the Effects of Policies

Organizations with health policy interests devote considerable attention to discerning the effects of policies. They do this because organizations are dynamic, open systems that exist in the context of a larger external environment and engage in ongoing exchanges with others in their external environments, including exchanges with the participants in the policymaking process. Organizations are influenced, sometimes dramatically, by what happens in their external environments.

The primary process organizations employ to discern important information in their environments is called *environmental scanning* (Duncan, Ginter, and Swayne 1992). Those who do this well make discernments about relevant policies accurately, and often in advance of their impacts.

The scanning process, which is illustrated in Figure 6.2, provides a "lens" through which an organization can see, or discern, that specific information in its environment that it should be aware of. Policies and the circumstances and issues surrounding them are one such type of information. But other types of information, such as information about biological, cultural, demographic, ecological, economic, ethical, legal, political, psychological, social, and technological factors, can also be quite important. Organizations scan their external environments for a wide variety of information, including information about policies.

The scanning process includes more than merely discerning important information. It also includes organizing the information in useful ways and evaluating the information in order to plot the issues that are likely to impact on the organization. In doing this, scanning becomes a process of forecasting. The end result of effective environmental scanning is the full discernment and understanding of policy-related information that might impact on the organization.

Influencing Policies

In addition to their organizational commitments to discerning relevant information about the policies that might affect them, organizations that are impacted by health policies also develop strong operational commitments to devising ways to influence these policies, both in their formulation and in their implementation. There is nothing innately wrong with this operational objective, although it goes almost without saying that the process can easily be tainted by overzealous attempts to influence policies for self-serving purposes.

Organizations have available to them two principal methods of influencing policies. They can present and push their views, often through an association or interest group and often in the form of lobbying, in an effort to have their views influence policies. They can also seek to influence policies by filing lawsuits in which they challenge certain policies or certain aspects of the implementation of policies. When a policy is being challenged in this way, it is common for organizations or associations with some interest in the issue to submit legal briefs as friends of the court (amicus curiae).

Figure 6.2 The Concept of Scanning an Organization's External
Environment

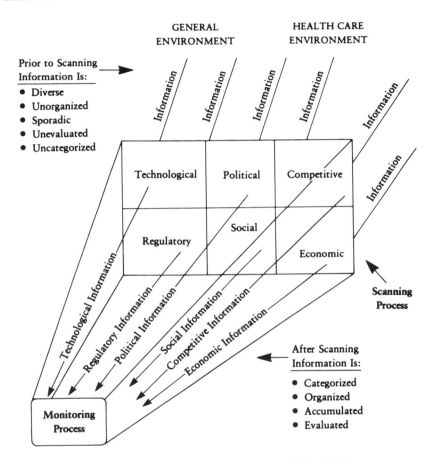

SCANNING AS THE ORGANIZATION'S LENS

The scanning process allows the organization to focus on technological, political, competitive, regulatory, social and economic issues, trends, dilemmas, and events important to the organization. The "viewing process" must sort diverse, unorganized information. This process also filters out information not relevant to the mission of the organization.

Reprinted with permission by PWS-Kent Publishing, as it appeared in W. J. Duncan, P. M. Ginter, and L. E. Swayne, *Strategic Management of Health Care Organizations*, Boston: PWS-Kent Publishing Company, p. 87. © 1992.

Influence on policies is exerted at several points in the policy-making process depicted earlier in Figures 2.1, 3.1, 4.1, and 5.1. Organizations, especially associations representing their constituent member organizations (e.g., the AHA, the AMA, or the AARP), can help establish the policy agenda by the submission of information about problems and possible solutions. They can and often do participate in the actual drafting of proposed legislation and are frequent participants in the hearings associated with the development of legislation.

Influence can also be exerted in the rulemaking stage where regulations that are to be used to guide the implementation of policies are written. At this stage of the policymaking process, especially, the provision of information based on operating experience can be influential. Wise policymakers, of course, realize that organizations and their lobbyists present information in ways that are self-serving. However, the information is still useful and can be influential. Policymakers are quite willing to receive and consider information from organizations that will be affected by policies. In fact, rulemaking, at the federal level, which mandates a notice of proposed rulemaking and the issuance of proposed regulations *before* final regulations can be adopted, is intentionally designed to facilitate the active participation of interested and affected parties. Activities preceding the writing of final regulations explicitly permit interested parties to comment on proposed regulations and to offer suggestions about their final form. Organizations that may be affected by policies, and the regulations under which they are implemented, are well advised to use this public comment period as an opportune time to influence policies.

One of the more pervasive strategies that organizations have adopted in their efforts to influence policies that might affect them is participation in political action committees, or PACs. As Table 6.1 shows, a number of organizations with health policy interests make sizable campaign contributions to policymakers through participation in PACs. PACs facilitate the aggregation and targeting of contributions. Few believe that PAC contributions directly influence many policy decisions; however, it is widely acknowledged that they help ensure access to policymakers (Rakich, Longest, and Darr 1992).

The use of the nation's courts, both state and federal, as a means to influence health policies is increasing. As was discussed in Chapter 5, in recent years the courts have influenced health policies heavily in four relatively new areas: the coverage decisions made by insurers in both the private and public sectors, the Medicaid program's payment rates to hospitals and nursing homes, the antitrust issues involved in hospital mergers, and issues related to the charitable mission and tax-exempt status of nonprofit hospitals (Anderson 1992).

Table 6.1   Top 20 Health PACs in 1992

Political Action Committees	*Total Contributions*
American Medical Association	$3,237,153
American Dental Association	1,434,408
American Academy of Ophthalmology	801,527
American Chiropractic Association	657,846
American Hospital Association	507,538
American Podiatry Association	401,000
American Optometric Association	398,366
American Health Care Association	382,019
American College of Emergency Physicians	330,725
American Nurses Association	306,519
Association for the Advancement of Psychology	273,743
American Physical Therapy Association	198,941
Eli Lilly & Company	195,530
Pfizer Inc.	188,100
Schering-Plough Corporation	186,050
Federation of American Health Systems	180,350
Glaxo Inc.	175,522
American Psychiatric Association	165,980
American Association of Oral & Maxillofacial Surgery	163,000
Abbott Laboratories	157,075

Source: Data from the Center for Responsive Politics, as cited in "Health Groups Shop for Reform with Big Political Contributions," *Journal of American Health Policy* 3, no. 4 (July–August 1993): 37–39.

The role of courts in the nation's social policy is by no means limited to health policy. In the past few decades the courts have been increasingly involved in influencing policies in areas such as school desegregation, the environment, and prison reform. Kagan (1991), among others, argues that the courts, as a means of influencing policies, provide a number of specific advantages: promoting minority rights, assuring more humane conditions in government institutions such as mental hospitals, and appropriately restraining bureaucratic arbitrariness.

In addition, utilizing the courts provides one very important structural advantage to organizations seeking to influence policies through litigation—the court's ability, indeed its requirement, to focus narrowly on the issues involved in a specific case. The organization initiating a court case has the opportunity to control, to a large extent, the issues to be addressed and to have its side of the issues receive detailed attention. This stands in stark contrast to the wide open—if not chaotic—political arena in which most efforts to influence policies must occur.

Horowitz (1977), among others, however, has expressed concern over courts' limitations in influencing policies. One limitation is particularly relevant to the issue of the use of the courts by organizations attempting to exert influence on policies—that is, the lack of appropriate educational background or experience that would prepare most judges to be able to evaluate critically the technical information necessary to resolve complex social policy issues. As has been pointed out regarding this limitation:

> Unlike in the legislative or executive branches, in which policymakers can develop expertise in a specific substantive area over a period of years, judges usually have to be educated on a particular issue at the beginning of each trial. Critics of the judicial process also have noted that much of the information can be filtered by the litigation process and that certain information can be stifled by the adversarial system if one side is able to withold or successfully prevent the introduction of specific data. (Anderson 1992, 97)

Limitations aside, courts are increasingly involved in health policymaking. We can reasonably anticipate that organizations will continue to avail themselves of this means of influencing the policies that affect them. In fact, the use of this mechanism is likely to increase as health policies become more numerous, complex, and important to the ultimate performance of many types of organizations.

Conclusion

Policies that result from the highly complex, interactive, and cyclical health policymaking process have outcomes and consequences that are perceived and felt by individuals, groups of individuals, and organizations. Those who are affected share two fundamental concerns about the process: discerning the potential impact of policies on themselves and influencing the formulation, implementation, and modification of these policies.

Effective discernment and influencing abilities usually rely on the pooled resources that can be made available only through organizations. This is why the consideration of the impact of policies on people is, for the most part, best made by consideration of the impact on organizations and the organizations' responsive efforts to discern impact and their corollory efforts to influence policies.

Discernment is accomplished through environmental scanning. This scanning provides a "window" through which an organization can see information about policies and their potential impact. Through effective environmental scanning, organizations process information so that it can be used to plot the issues that are likely to impact on them. In so doing, scanning turns into a process of forecasting. When the process is successful, organizations discern the potential effect of policies.

Organizations seek to influence policies so that their impact will be more favorable—or, at least, less harmful—to them. Two approaches to influencing policies are widely used by organizations: (1) they present their views, often through an association or interest group, at many points in the policymaking process so that their views can be considered in the making of policies; or (2) they influence policies through bringing lawsuits to challenge certain policies or their implementation.

References

Anderson, G. F. "The Courts and Health Policy: Strengths and Limitations." *Health Affairs* 11, no. 4 (Winter 1992): 95–109.

Burner, S. T., D. R. Waldo, and D. R. McKusick. "National Health Expenditures Projections Through 2030." *Health Care Financing Review* 14, no. 1 (Fall 1992): 1–29.

Crane, S. C., A. S. Hersh, and S. M. Shortell. "Challenges for Health Services Research in the 1990s." In *Improving Health Policy and Management: Nine Critical Research Issues for the 1990s*, edited by S. M. Shortell and U. E. Reinhardt, 369–84. Ann Arbor, MI: Health Administration Press, 1992.

Cummings, K. C., and R. M. Abell. "Losing Sight of the Shore: How a Future Integrated American Health Care Organization Might Look." *Health Care Management Review* 18, no. 2 (Spring 1993): 39–50.

De Lew, N., G. Greenberg, and K. Kinchen. "A Layman's Guide to the U.S. Health Care System." *Health Care Financing Review* 14, no. 1 (Fall 1992): 151–69.

Duncan, W. J., P. M. Ginter, and L. E. Swayne. *Strategic Management of Health Care Organizations*. Boston: PWS-Kent Publishing Company, 1992.

Durenberger, D., and S. B. Foote. "Medical Technology Meets Managed Competition." *Journal of American Health Policy* 3, no. 3 (May–June 1993): 23–28.

Employee Benefit Research Institute. *Issue Brief, No. 118*. Washington, DC: The Institute, 1991.

Health Insurance Association of America. *The Health Insurance Industry Strategy for Containing Health Care Costs*. Washington, DC: The Association, 1990.

Horowitz, D. L. *The Courts and Social Policy*. Washington, DC: The Brookings Institution, 1977.

Joint Commission on Accreditation of Healthcare Organizations. *Committed To Quality: An Introduction to the Joint Commission on Accreditation of Healthcare Organizations*. Oakbrook Terrace, IL: The Commission, 1990.

Kagan, R.A. "Adversarial Legalism and American Government." *Journal of Policy Analysis and Management* 10, no. 3 (Summer 1991): 369–406.

Koch, A. L. "Financing Health Services." In *Introduction to Health Services*, 4th ed., edited by S. J. Williams and P. R. Torrens, 299–331. Albany, NY: Delmar Publishers Inc., 1993.

Longest, B. B., Jr., and T. Detre. "A Cost-Containment Agenda for Academic Health Centers." *Hospital & Health Services Administration* 36, no. 1 (Spring 1991): 77–93.

Mick, S. S., and D. A. Conrad. "The Decision to Integrate Vertically in Health Care Organizations." *Hospital & Health Services Administration* 33, no. 3 (Fall 1988): 345–60.

Mick, S. S., and I. Moscovice. "Health Care Professionals." In *Introduction to Health Services*, 4th ed., edited by S. J. Williams and P. R. Torrens, 269–96. Albany, NY: Delmar Publishers Inc., 1993.

National League for Nursing. *Nursing Data Source 1991*, Vol. I. New York: The League, 1991.

Pickett, G. E., and J. J. Hanlon. *Public Health Administration and Practice*, 9th ed. St. Louis, MO: Times Mirror/Mosby College Publishing, 1990.

Rakich, J. S., B. B. Longest, Jr., and K. Darr. *Managing Health Services Organizations*, 3rd ed. Baltimore, MD: Health Professions Press, 1992.

Shugars, D. A., E. H. O'Neil, and J.D. Bader, editors. *Healthy America: Practitioners for 2005, An Agenda for Action for U.S. Health Professional Schools.* Durham, NC: The Pew Health Professions Commission, 1991.

U.S. Congressional Budget Office. *Economic Implications of Rising Health Care Costs.* Washington, DC: U.S. Government Printing Office, 1992.

————. *Rising Health Care Costs: Causes, Implications, and Strategies.* Washington, DC: U.S. Government Printing Office, 1991.

U.S. Department of Commerce. *U.S. Industrial Outlook, 1993.* Washington, DC: U.S. Government Printing Office, 1993.

Figure 7.1 A Model of the Public Policymaking Process in the United States: The Synthesis

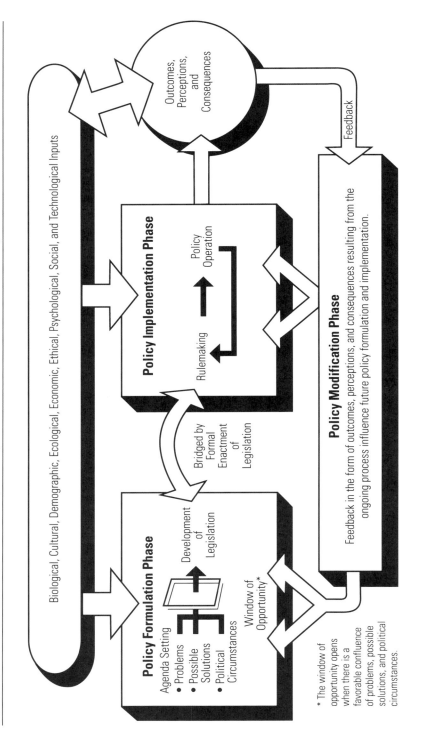

7

Synthesizing the Policymaking Process

$\mathbf{H}$ealth, defined positively and broadly, is the maximization of the biological and clinical indicators of organ function and the maximization of physical, mental, and role functioning in everyday life. Thought of in this way, health can be pursued through proactive interventions aimed at many factors that affect health. As we have seen, health determinants include the physical, sociocultural, and economic environments in which people live; their lifestyles and behaviors; their heredity; and the type, quality, and timing of health care services that people receive.

Given the innate desirability of health and the important role that the pursuit of health plays in the nation's economy, it is not at all surprising that government, at all levels, is keenly interested in health affairs. This interest drives public policymaking related to health. Like public policies in other domains, such as the economy, education, or social welfare, health policies are authoritative decisions made in the legislative, executive, or judicial branches of government that are intended to direct or influence the actions, behaviors, or decisions of others. The fact that they pertain to our pursuit of health makes them health policies.

In the United States, health policies are made through a dynamic public policymaking process involving the interactive participation of many members of the health policy community in several interconnected and interdependent phases of activities. This chapter will briefly synthesize what has been discussed in earlier chapters about this process and will conclude with a discussion of three factors that I believe will exert especially potent influence on the way this process operates—and on its outcomes and consequences—in the years immediately ahead.

Policy Formulation, Implementation, and Modification: The Interconnection

The process through which health policy is made in the United States has grown in importance as an element of American political life during the second half of the twentieth century. This has occurred because both society's expectations regarding health and the costs of pursuing these expectations have risen dramatically. There are many reasons to think that the evolving results of this process will continue to be critically important to the American people and to their policymakers for the foreseeable future.

Figure 7.1 is a schematic of the process that we have used throughout the book. One important feature of the process—a feature that can be better emphasized now that each phase of the process has been discussed at some length in previous chapters—is how tightly interconnected the phases of the policymaking process are. The phases do not unfold in neat sequence. Instead, they blend together in a gestalt of actors and actions that yield policies. Figure 7.2 illustrates the closely intertwined relationships among the formulation, implementation, and modification phases of policymaking.

While both figures reflect the distinctly cyclical character of the policymaking process in its operation, Figure 7.2 emphasizes this especially strongly, demonstrating that the cycle of public policymaking is an ongoing phenomenon, one without definitive beginnings or endings.

The model of health policymaking presented in this book also emphasizes that the process is heavily influenced by factors external to the process itself. Such influences are biological, cultural, demographic, ecological, economic, ethical, psychological, social, and technological factors. Conceptualizing the process through which health policies are made as the dynamic and interrelated phases of activities—formulation, implementation, and modification—contained in this model offers students of the process, as well as participants in the process, a vehicle to better appreciate both its full dimensions and complexity.

In this comprehensive model of policymaking, policy formulation incorporates activities associated with agenda setting and subsequently with the development of legislation. Policy implementation incorporates activities associated with rulemaking and policy operation. Policy modification exists as the third phase in the process because perfection cannot be achieved in the other two phases and because policies are established and exist in a dynamic world. Policies suitable for today's circumstances may become archaic and inadequate tomorrow.

The formulation phase (making the decisions that lead to policies) and the implementation phase (taking actions and making additional

Figure 7.2   The Intertwined Relationships Among Policy Formulation, Implementation, and Modification

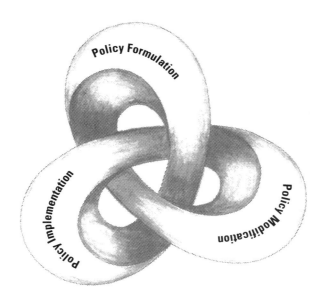

decisions necessary to implement policies) are bridged by the formal enactment of legislation. Once enacted as laws, policies must still be implemented if they are to have an impact. Responsibility for this rests predominantly with the executive branch departments and agencies, entities that exist primarily to implement the policies embodied in legislation.

But it is important to remember that some of the implementation decisions made within the implementing organizations themselves become policies. Rules and regulations promulgated in order to implement a law are policies just as are the laws whose implementation the rules support. Similarly, judicial decisions regarding the applicability of laws to specific situations or regarding the appropriateness of the actions of implementing organizations are decisions that are included in the nation's health policy.

Policy modification, which is shown as a feedback loop in Figure 7.1, can range from minor alterations in the operation of policies to changes in the rules and regulations used to implement policies, to modest amendments to existing legislation, to fundamental policy changes. In the latter case, the outcomes and consequences of implementing certain policies feed back to the agenda-setting stage of the process. For example, the challenges of formulating policies to contain health care costs that face policymakers in the 1990s are in part a consequence of the success of previous policies such as those that expanded access or subsidized an increased supply of human resources and advanced technologies to be used in the pursuit of health. The outcomes and consequences of these and other prior policies strongly influence contemporary policymaking. But there are some other important influences on this process as well.

Critical Influences on Health Policymaking in the United States

There are three especially potent influences on the policymaking process that will help shape American health policy in the years ahead. They are the nature of the goals and objectives to which health policy will be directed; the nature of the political marketplace in which health policy will be made; and the looming reality that decisions about health policy must, ultimately, be made under the constraints of economic scarcity.

The goals and objectives of health policy

Some relationships in our complex world are so simple that we have a tendency to overlook them. One of these is the correlation between policy objectives and policies. Policies are developed to achieve policy objectives. This relationship, in and of itself, makes no assumptions about either the appropriateness or the attainability of objectives; it merely recognizes the innate relationship between objectives and the policies that are intended to achieve them (Longest 1988). But this simple relationship is extremely important to the nature of future health policy: The objectives toward which health policies will be directed will, perhaps more than anything else, help shape future policies.

There are many alternative objectives to which past health policies have been directed; we have the same set of potential objectives to guide future policies. As we have seen, health in human beings is a function of a number of interrelated variables, including the environment in which people live, their choices about lifestyle and behavior, their genetic histories, and the health care services to which they have access. Because so many variables affect health, we have developed a multitude, essentially an unranked multitude, of health policy objectives in a variety of areas.

Under the broad rubric of the nation's health policy objectives is the intermingling of objectives pertaining to: improving access to, reducing the costs of, and increasing the quality of personal health services; removing from the environment substances and conditions that have a negative impact on health; advancing the scientific and technological base of our pursuit of health; improving the housing and living conditions of our citizens; improving the economic circumstances of citizens; making citizens more safety conscious on highways and in other dangerous places; improving the nutrition of citizens; moderating citizens' consumption of food, drink, and chemicals; and modifying citizens' sexual behaviors. Coupled with our persistent concern about how to pay for achieving any and all of these objectives, this plethora of objectives has stimulated a vast montage of poorly integrated—sometimes even conflicting—policies intended to meet the objectives, although not necessarily in any particular order.

So long as the objectives for health policy continue to be established in piecemeal fashion, the policies intended to realize the objectives will be piecemeal and disjointed. We are making some progress in rationalizing and clarifying some of our health policy objectives. Under the stimulus of the Clinton administration's commitment to health reform in the early 1990s, for example, the nation is finally making progress toward establishing a clear-cut objective for cost reduction in the health care system (i.e., to bring growth in health care costs in line with growth in GDP). Similarly, a clear objective may soon emerge to guarantee comprehensive health coverage for all Americans as part of the nation's health policy. These are important steps in the direction of rationalizing our health policy objectives. But they should not be mistaken for the establishment of a comprehensive and integrated set of health policy objectives for the nation. This larger, more difficult, and much more important task still awaits our health policymakers. And it will require extraordinarily broad thinking.

Broad thinking, an inherently difficult task, is made even more so in regard to health policy by the focusing effect of the interest groups who seek to influence policymakers' thinking and actions so that they reflect particular interests and preferences. The defining purpose of interest groups is, after all, to identify the interests, which tend to be narrow, of the group's members and to pursue these interests vigorously.

Broad thinking by health policymakers may also remain rare and elusive because of other structural characteristics of the American policymaking process. The process, as we have seen, has a number of features that work to splinter thinking and isolate decisions rather than to stimulate comprehensive visions of where policies should lead the nation and to orchestrate the integrated set of decisions needed to realize the vision.

The inchoate steps at health reform initiated by the Clinton administration are a laudable beginning toward the needed broader thinking regarding health policy. But it should escape no one that the primary focus of these efforts is on reform of the way we organize and finance *health care services*—services that as we have seen, only play a part in society's larger pursuit of health. Truly expansive health reform thinking would incorporate attention to the physical, social, and economic environments in which people live and give more attention to their lifestyles and heredity as important determinants of their health. It would not rely so disproportionately on evening out access to health care services, although this is an important component of an effective national health policy.

The political marketplace

The policymaking process occurs within the context of a political marketplace, where many participants seek to further their own interests. This fact, which is unlikely to change, will continue to exert significant influence on the shape of the nation's health policy. The interests of the participants in the political market for health policies include not only self-interests, such as some economic or political advantage, but they also include the public interest; at least they include certain participants' perceptions of what is best for the nation.

Policies have value in this political marketplace. Both suppliers and demanders of policies recognize their innate value, and both stand to reap benefits and incur costs because of policies. Any individual can, at least theoretically, be a demander of policies. However, as we have seen, the ratio of costs to benefits for individuals limits the extent to which citizen-demanders participate in the political markets for policies, at least as individuals. Instead, well-organized interest groups tend to be the most effective demanders of policies. Their effectiveness is obtained by combining and concentrating the resources of the members of the group to change the ratio between the costs and benefits of participation.

Members of the legislative, executive, and judicial branches of government play roles as suppliers of policies, although the roles are played in different ways. Members of the legislative branch supply policies in the form of statutes or laws and programs. They make calculations about the benefits and costs, and to whom, of their policymaking decisions, and, factoring in the interests they choose to serve, make their decisions accordingly.

Members of the executive branch also play important roles as suppliers of policies. They propose policies in the form of statutes or programs and seek to influence legislators to enact their preferred policies. The hierarchical executive branch of government, including chief and top-level executives as well as executives and managers in charge of departments and agencies of government, makes policies in the form of rules and regulations used to implement statutes and programs. In this, they are direct suppliers of policies. Elected and appointed executives and managers are joined in the rulemaking role by career bureaucrats who thus also become suppliers of policies in the political marketplace.

Finally, the judicial branch also is an important supplier of policies. The courts are involved in numerous and diverse areas of health policy: termination of treatment, environmental responsibilities, approval of new drugs, mental health law, genetics, antitrust, and on and on. Whenever a court interprets an ambiguous statute, establishes judicial procedure, or interprets the U.S. Constitution, it makes policies. These activities do not differ conceptually from legislators enacting statutes or members of the executive branch establishing rules and regulations for the implementation of the statutes. The authoritative decisions intended to influence others that result from all three activities are policies.

The health policy domain includes a rich set of stakeholders, some of whom demand policies while others supply them. The policy community formed by these demanders and suppliers of health policies has undergone dramatic changes as the twentieth century has unfolded. Today, this community is heterogeneous and loosely structured; its members compete with each other, often fiercely, over the optimal design of the nation's health policy.

Relationships among participants in the health policy community are more fluid and unstable than they have ever been before. This circumstance shows no signs of abating as the participants face an evolving set of relationships that will be forged in the pressure and heat of health care reform in the years ahead. The fluidity and instability of these relationships makes it difficult for the suppliers of health policies to discern what the demanders really want. Or, more accurately, it makes it difficult for the suppliers to decide which of the diverse demands they should attempt to meet. This, in turn, makes it very difficult to predict the path of the nation's health policy. But we can be certain that the eventual reconfiguration among participants in the health policy community will help shape policy, just as the configurations among these participants have been extremely influential in the past.

The looming reality of economic scarcity

A final noteworthy influence on American health policymaking, one that will affect future policymaking dramatically, is the fact that health policy decisions must eventually be made within the context of economic scarcity. In a context where scarcity is recognized, limited resources will be seen to have alternative uses and people will be seen to have a variety of preferences about how the resources should be used. Victor Fuchs (1974), with elegance and prescience, warned us two decades ago about the ultimate necessity of making some difficult choices about health: "We cannot have all the health or all the medical care that we would like to have" (7). Others have echoed and extended this warning (Aaron and Schwartz 1984; Callahan 1987).

But, even now, many members of the health policy community appear able to ignore the fact that we do not have sufficient resources to provide all the support that people want in their pursuit of health, at least not if their other wants are to be simultaneously met as well. There is no reason to think that our wants regarding health will abate in the future, nor any reason to anticipate that some large new pool of resources to pay for them will be found.

Our health policy history to date has shown that ignoring the reality of economic scarcity permits people to ignore the consequent necessity to make difficult choices about the allocation of scarce resources. But society ultimately faces incredibly difficult choices about its pursuit of health, both in terms of its allocations to the various determinants of health and vis-à-vis other, non-health wants.

Already, we know many of the important questions regarding this issue. The most familiar ones include: Are scarce resources better utilized at the beginning or end of life? Are 25,000 vaccinations better than a single organ transplant? Is society better served by more physicians or more teachers? engineers? or musicians? Is it better served by more museums, art galleries, playgrounds, or stock car racing tracks than by more hospitals? Is it better to clean up the environment or to find better ways of treating asthma and lung cancer? We do not know the answers to such questions, and we do not even know the criteria to use in answering the questions. Are the criteria to be ethical or economic? Should they be both? In what mix?

The timing with which future policymakers turn their attention to such questions is unpredictable. The only certainty is that sooner or later they must address them in the context of the nation's health policy. But three categories of past and contemporary participants in health policymaking impede our ability to reflect the reality of scarcity in our policymaking. They appear especially unable or unwilling to accept that we face a growing challenge to allocate the resources devoted to the pursuit of health through a series of painfully difficult social choices.

The first category are the *romantics*. These are the people who do not recognize the reality of scarcity. Such people do not believe that society's resources are so scarce as to preclude the simultaneous fulfillment of all that its members might want in their pursuit of health *and* to satisfy their other wants. In their view instead, poor planning, greed, injustice, or some other scapegoat is responsible for the fact that we must make choices about resource allocation. Because the romantics deny the inevitability of difficult resource allocation choices, they impede society's progress toward making the choices.

There is an important subcategory of romantics that we can call the *pseudo-romantics*. These people actually recognize the innate reality of economic scarcity, but, usually for political reasons, choose to deny that scarcity is a reality to be dealt with. Such people, in order to have their way, deny scarcity, often relying on the possibility that someone else will give something up so that their preferences can be realized, or that new resources will be found. The pseudo-romantics tend to be people who want to serve the public interest, but who are unwilling to acknowledge that all benefits must eventually be paid for. The pseudo-romantics also impede society's ability to make its resource allocation choices optimally, but for a different reason than that afflicting the real romantics.

The second distinct category of people who make it difficult for the nation to make the ultimately necessary painful choices about health policy, choices that fully reflect the realities of economic scarcity, are the *truly self-serving*. Such people may know very well about the reality of economic scarcity, but they are so intent on making certain that their interests are served in policymaking that they will ignore the reality of scarcity. In this they are like the pseudo-romantics. But for the truly self-serving, the reason to ignore the scarcity issue is selfish; for the pseudo-romantics it may be for some larger public-interest purpose.

The truly self-serving tend to be so intent on making certain that their interests are served that other issues become secondary. The larger picture dictated by a concern about the reality of economic scarcity does not matter very much to people in the truly self-serving category. Truly self-serving participants have been well represented in past policymaking for health and will likely continue to impede the ability of society to make health policy decisions that fully recognize the constraints imposed by scarcity.

The third category of people in the health policy community who impede progress toward fully integrating the reality of economic scarcity into the nation's health policy are the *procrastinators*. This category includes people who accept the ultimate reality of economic scarcity and even accept that it requires difficult allocation choices, but who believe that the fateful day when scarcity must actually guide decisions can be postponed still further. Procrastinators accept the fact that, ultimately, economic scarcity will very heavily influence American health policy. But, in their view, we in the United States can continue to postpone these difficult decisions. For the procrastinators, the difficult societal decisions about resource allocation for the pursuit of health can be left to future decision makers.

Figure 7.3   Health's Historical Share of the Nation's GDP

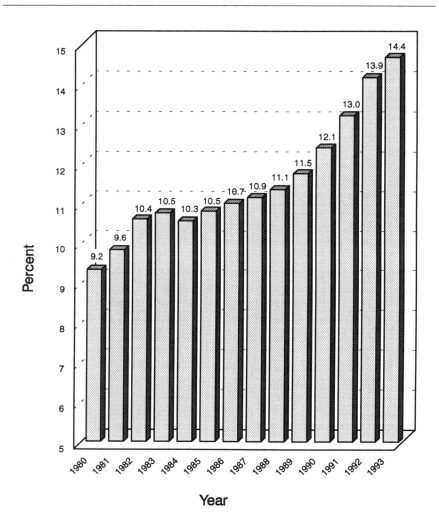

So far, the procastinators have been right. It has indeed been possible to postpone dealing with the reality of scarcity in the nation's health policy. One need only look at the pattern of steady growth in the share of the nation's GDP devoted to health care shown in Figure 7.3 to verify this fact (Schieber, Poullier, and Greenwald 1992).

Figure 7.4   Health's Projected Share of the Nation's GDP

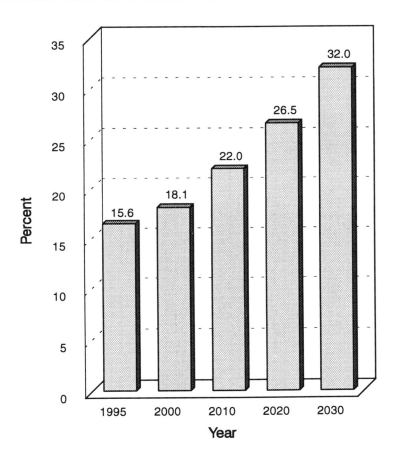

However, projection of this statistic based on continuation of *current* policies suggests that procrastination on this issue does indeed have a finite life, as shown in Figure 7.4 (Burner, Waldo, and McKusick 1992).

The challenges inherent in the broad thinking that must eventually underlie a complete calculus of optimal health policy for the United States are daunting. Ultimately, our health policy must more fully reflect the constraints imposed by economic scarcity. And, invariably, this policy will be made within the context of a volatile political marketplace. These facts cause legitimate concern about our abilities to make health policy that will best support our citizenry's quest for health. Yet, this quest is so fundamental to our society's well-being and to the well-being of each of its members that the goal of an optimal health policy must be pursued as vigorously as any national goal we establish. Knowledge of the process by which such a policy might be made and an informed appreciation of the intricacies of the process are powerful allies in attempts to influence—or just to understand—America's health policy.

References

Aaron, H. J., and W. B. Schwartz. *The Painful Prescription: Rationing Hospital Care.* Washington, DC: The Brookings Institution, 1984.

Burner, S. T., D. R. Waldo, and D. R. McKusick. "National Health Expenditures Projections Through 2030." *Health Care Financing Review* 14, no. 1 (Fall 1992): 1–29.

Callahan, D. *Setting Limits: Medical Goals in an Aging Society.* New York: Simon and Schuster, 1987.

Fuchs, V. R. *Who Shall Live?* New York: Basic Books, Inc., 1974.

Longest, B. B., Jr. "American Health Policy in the Year 2000." *Hospital & Health Services Administration* 33, no. 4 (Winter 1988): 419–34.

Schieber, G. J., J. P. Poullier, and L. M. Greenwald. "U.S. Health Expenditure Performance: An International Comparison and Data Update." *Health Care Financing Review* 13, no. 4 (Summer 1992): 1–87.

Appendix

Chronological List of Selected U.S. Federal Laws Pertaining to Health

1798

An act of 16 July, passed by the Fifth Congress of the United States, taxed the employers of merchant seamen to fund arrangements for their health care through the Marine Hospital Service. In the language of the act, "the master or owner of every ship or vessel of the United States arriving from a foreign port into any port in the United States shall . . . render to the collector a true account of the number of seamen that shall have been employed on board such vessel . . . and shall pay to the said collector, at the rate of twenty cents per month, for every seaman so employed . . . . " The act stipulated in Section 2 that "the President of the United States is hereby authorized, out of the same, to provide for the temporary relief and maintenance of sick or disabled seamen in the hospitals, or other proper institutions now established in the several ports . . . . "

1882

An act of 3 August, was the nation's first general immigration law and included the first federal medical excludability provisions affecting those who wished to immigrate to the United States. The act authorized state officials to board arriving ships to examine the condition of passengers. In the language of the act, "if on such examination, there shall be found among such passengers any convict, lunatic, idiot, or any person unable to take care of himself or herself without becoming a public charge, . . . such persons shall not be permitted to land."

1891

An act of 3 March, added the phrase, "persons suffering from a loathsome or a contagious disease" to the list of medical excludability criteria for people seeking to immigrate to the United States.

1902

P.L. 57-244,* the *Biologics Control Act*, was the first federal law regulating the interstate and foreign sale of biologics (viruses, serums, toxins, and analogous products). The law established a national board and gave its members authority to establish regulations for licensing producers of biologics.

1906

P.L. 59-384, the *Pure Food and Drug Act* (or the Wiley Act), defined adulterated and mislabeled foods and drugs and prohibited their transport in interstate commerce. Passage of this legislation followed several years of intense campaigning by reformers and extensive newspaper coverage of examples of unwholesome and adulterated foods and of the widespread use of ineffective patent medicines.

1920

P.L. 66-141, the *Snyder Act*, was the first federal legislation pertaining to health care for Native Americans. Prior to the passage of this legislation, there were some health-related provisions in treaties between the government and the Native Americans, but this was the first formal legislation on the subject. The act provided for general assistance, directing "the Bureau of Indian Affairs, under the supervision of the Secretary of the Interior to direct, supervise, and expend such monies as Congress may from time to time appropriate, for the benefit, care, and assistance of the Indians throughout the United States . . . . "

1921

P.L. 67-97, the *Maternity and Infancy Act* (or the Sheppard-Towner Act), provided grants to states to help them develop health services for mothers and their children. The law was allowed to lapse in 1929, although it has served as a prototype for federal grants-in-aid to the states.

1935

P.L. 74-271, the *Social Security Act*, a landmark law developed and passed during the Great Depression, established the "Social Security" program of old age ben-

---

* Reflecting the convention adopted by the Congress, acts began to be referred to by their public law numbers. These numbers reflect both the number of the enacting Congress and the sequence in which the laws were enacted. For example, Public Law (P.L.) 57-244 means the 244th law passed by the 57th Congress. Hereafter, the public law numbers of health-related federal laws in this chronology are provided.

efits. The legislation also included provisions for other benefits such as federal financial assistance to the states for their public assistance programs for the needy elderly, dependent children, and the blind. This legislation also provided incentives for the establishment of state unemployment funds and provided financial assistance for maternal and child health and child welfare services and significantly increased federal assistance for state and local public health programs.

1936

P.L. 74-846, the *Walsh-Healy Act*, authorized federal regulation of industrial safety in companies doing business with the U.S. government.

1937

P.L. 75-244, the *National Cancer Institute Act*, established the first categorical institute within the National Institute of Health, which had been created in 1930 to serve as the administrative home for the research conducted by the U.S. Public Health Service.

1938

P.L. 75-540, the *LaFollette-Bulwinkle Act*, provided grants-in-aid to the states to support their investigation and control of venereal disease.

P.L. 75-717, the *Food, Drug and Cosmetic Act*, extended federal authority to ban new drugs from the market until they were approved by the Food and Drug Administration.

1939

P.L. 76-19, the *Reorganization Act*, transferred the Public Health Service from the Treasury Department to the new Federal Security Agency (FSA). In 1953 the FSA was transformed into the U.S. Department of Health, Education and Welfare (DHEW) that, with the subsequent establishment of a new cabinet level Department of Education in 1980, was itself transformed into the U.S. Department of Health and Human Services (DHHS).

1941

P.L. 77-146, the *Nurse Training Act*, provided schools of nursing with support to permit them to increase enrollments and improve their physical facilities.

1944

P.L. 78-410, the *Public Health Service Act*, revised and consolidated in one place all existing legislation pertaining to the U.S. Public Health Service. The legislation provided for the organization, staffing, and functions and activities of the Public Health Service. This law has subsequently been utilized as a vehicle, through amendments to the legislation, for a number of important federal grant-in-aid programs.

1945

P.L. 79-15, the *McCarran-Ferguson Act*, expressly exempted the "business of insurance" from federal antitrust legislation (the Sherman Antritrust Act of 1890, the Clayton Act of 1914, and the Federal Trade Commission Act of 1914) to the extent that insurance was regulated by state law and did not involve "acts of boycott, coercion, or intimidation." A significant part of the underlying reasoning Congress used in exempting insurance, including health insurance, was the view that the determination of underwriting risks would require the cooperation and sharing of information among competing insurance companies.

1946

P.L. 79-487, the *National Mental Health Act*, authorized extensive federal support for mental health research and treatment programs and established grants-in-aid to the states for their mental health activities. The legislation also transformed the Public Health Services's Division of Mental Health into the National Institute of Mental Health.

P.L. 79-725, the *Hospital Survey and Construction Act* (or the Hill-Burton Act), was "An Act to amend the Public Health Service Act [see the 1944 P.L. 78-410] to authorize grants to the States for surveying their hospital and public health centers and for planning construction of additional facilities, and to authorize grants to assist in such construction." The legislation was enacted because Congress recognized a widespread shortage of hospital facilities (few were built during the Great Depression and World War II). Under provisions of the act, the states were required to submit a state plan for the construction of hospital facilities based on a survey of need to receive federal funds, which could be dispersed for projects within states.

1948

P.L. 80-655, the *National Health Act*, pluralized the NIH by establishing a second categorical institute, the National Heart Institute. Hereafter, the NIH became the National Institutes of Health.

P.L. 80-845, the *Water Pollution Control Act*, was enacted, in part, "in consequence of the benefits to the public health and welfare by the abatement of stream pollution . . . . " The act left the primary responsibility for water pollution control with the states.

1952

P.L. 82-414, the *Immigration and Nationality Act* (or the McCarran-Walter Act), followed an extensive study by the Congress of immigration policy and practice. Among the law's provisions were a number of modifications in the medical excludability scheme affecting people wishing to immigrate to the United States. The act contained extensive provisions for observation and examination of aliens for the purpose of determining if they should be excluded for any of a number of specified "diseases or mental or physical defects or disabilities."

1954

P.L. 83-482, the *Medical Facilities Survey and Construction Act*, amended the Hill-Burton Act (see the 1946 P.L. 79-725) to greatly expand the Hill-Burton program's scope. The legislation authorized grants for surveys and construction of diagnostic and treatment centers (including hospital outpatient departments), chronic disease hospitals, rehabilitation facilities, and nursing homes.

P.L. 83-703, the *Atomic Energy Act*, established the Atomic Energy Commission and authorized it to license the use of atomic material in medical care.

1955

P.L. 84-159, the *Air Pollution Control Act*, provided for a program of research and technical assistance related to air pollution control. The law was enacted, in part, "in recognition of the dangers to the public health and welfare . . . from air pollution . . . . "

P.L. 84-377, the *Polio Vaccination Assistance Act*, provided for federal assistance to states for the operation of their polio vaccination programs.

1956

P.L. 84-569, the *Dependents Medical Care Act*, established the Civilian Health and Medical Program of the Uniformed Services (CHAMPUS) for the dependents of military personnel.

P.L. 84-652, the *National Health Survey Act*, provided for the first system of regularly collected health-related data by the Public Health Service. This continuing process is called the Health Interview Survey and provides a national household interview study of illness, disability, and health services utilization of the U.S. population.

P.L. 84-660, the *Water Pollution Control Act Amendments of 1956*, amended the Water Pollution Control Act (see the 1948 P.L. 80-845) and provided for federal technical services and financial aid to the states and to municipalities in their efforts to prevent and control water pollution.

P.L. 84-911, the *Health Amendments Act*, amended the Public Health Service Act (see the 1944 P.L. 78-410) by initiating federal assistance for the education and training of health personnel. Specifically, the law authorized traineeships for public health personnel and for advanced training for nurses. This support has been gradually broadened and extended by subsequent legislation to many categories of health personnel.

1958

P.L. 85-544, *Grants-in-aid to Schools of Public Health*, established a program of formula grants to the nation's schools of public health.

P.L. 85-929, the *Food Additives Amendment*, amended the Food, Drug and Cosmetic Act (see the 1938 P.L. 75-717) to require premarketing clearance from the FDA for new food additives. The so-called Delaney Clause, after Representative James Delaney who sponsored the provison, stated that "no additive shall be deemed to be safe if it is found to induce cancer when injested by man or animal
. . . . "

1959

P.L. 86-121, the *Indian Sanitation Facilities Act*, provided for the Surgeon General to "construct, improve, extend, or otherwise provide and maintain, by contract or otherwise, essential sanitation facilities for Indian homes, communities, and lands . . . . "

P.L. 86-352, the *Federal Employees Health Benefits Act*, permitted Blue Cross to negotiate a contract with the Civil Service Commission to provide health insurance coverage for federal employees. The contract served as a prototype for Blue Cross's subsequent involvement in the Medicare and Medicaid programs as a fiscal intermediary.

1960

P.L. 86-778, the *Social Security Amendments* (or the Kerr-Mills Act), amended the Social Security Act (see the 1935 P.L. 74-271) to establish a new program of medical assistance for the aged. Through this program, the federal government provided aid to the states for payments for medical care for "medically indigent" persons who were 65 years of age or older. The Kerr-Mills program, as it was called, was the forerunner of the Medicaid program established later in 1965 (see P.L. 89-97).

1962

P.L. 87-692, the *Health Services for Agricultural Migratory Workers Act*, authorized federal grants to clinics serving migrant farm workers and their families.

P.L. 87-781, the *Drug Amendments* (or the Kefauver-Harris Amendments), amended the Food, Drug and Cosmetic Act (see the 1938 P.L. 75-717) to significantly strengthen the provisions related to the regulation of therapeutic drugs. The changes required improved manufacturing practices and procedures and evidence that new drugs proposed for marketing be effective as well as safe. These amendments followed widespread adverse publicity about the serious negative side-effects of the drug thalidomide.

1963

P.L. 88-129, the *Health Professions Educational Assistance Act*, inaugurated construction grants for teaching facilities that trained physicians, dentists, pharmacists, podiatrists, nurses, or professional public health personnel. The grants were made contingent on schools' increasing their first-year enrollments. The legislation also provided for student loans and scholarships.

P.L. 88-156, the *Maternal and Child Health and Mental Retardation Planning Amendments*, amended the Social Security Act (see the 1935 P.L. 74-271). The changes were intended "to assist states and communities in preventing and combating mental retardation through expansion and improvement of the maternal and child health and crippled children's programs, through provision of prenatal, maternity, and infant care for individuals with conditions associated with childbearing that may lead to mental retardation, and through planning for comprehensive action to combat mental retardation."

P.L. 88-164, the *Mental Retardation Facilities and Community Mental Health Centers Construction Act*, was intended "to provide assistance in combating mental retardation through grants for construction of research centers and grants for facilities for the mentally retarded and assistance in improving mental health through grants for construction of community mental health centers, and for other purposes."

P.L. 88-206, the *Clean Air Act*, authorized direct grants to states and local governments to assist in their air pollution control efforts. The law also established federal enforcement of interstate air pollution restrictions.

1964

P.L. 88-443, the *Hospital and Medical Facilities Amendments*, amended the Hill-Burton Act (see the 1946 P.L. 79-725) to specifically earmark grants for modernizing or replacing existing hospitals.

P.L. 88-452, the *Economic Opportunity Act*, sometimes referred to as the Antipoverty Program, was intended to "mobilize the human and financial resources of the nation to combat poverty in the United States." This broad legislation affected health in a number of ways as it sought to improve the economic and social conditions under which many people lived.

P.L. 88-581, the *Nurse Training Act*, added a new Title, VIII, to the Public Health Service Act (see the 1944 P.L. 78-410). The legislation authorized separate funding for construction grants to schools of nursing, including associate degree and diploma schools. The law also provided for project grants whereby schools of nursing could strengthen their academic programs and provided for the establishment of student loan funds at these schools.

1965

P.L. 89-4, the *Appalachian Redevelopment Act*, sought to promote the economic, physical, and social development of the Appalachian region. Provisions in the law facilitated a number of steps to achieve this purpose including the establishment of community health centers and training programs for health personnel.

P.L. 89-73, the *Older Americans Act*, established an Administration on Aging to administer, through state agencies on aging, programs for the elderly. The agenda for the joint efforts of the federal agency and the state agencies was detailed in ten specific objectives for the nation's older citizens, including several that were related to their health.

P.L. 89-92, the *Federal Cigarette Labeling and Advertising Act*, required that all cigarette packages sold in the United States bear the label, "Caution: Cigarette Smoking May be Hazardous to Your Health."

P.L. 89-97, the *Social Security Amendments of 1965*, a landmark in the nation's health policy, established two new titles to the Social Security Act (see the 1935 P.L. 74-271): (1) Title XVIII, Health Insurance for the Aged, or Medicare; and (2)

Title XIX, Grants to the States for Medical Assistance Programs, or Medicaid. Enactment of these amendments followed many years of often acrimonious congressional debate about government's role and responsibility regarding ensuring access to health services for the citizenry. This legislation was made possible by the landslide dimensions of Lyndon B. Johnson's 1964 election to the presidency and by the accompanying largest Democratic majority in Congress since 1934.

The congressional debate over the Medicare legislation was fueled by intense opposition to it in some quarters, especially by the American Medical Association. The nation had never seen so feverish a lobbying campaign as it was exposed to regarding the Medicare program. Among the many tactics in the campaign, perhaps none is more entertaining in hindsight and certainly few are more representative of the campaign's tone, than the fact that the AMA sent every physician's spouse a recording to play in attempting to encourage their friends to write their representatives in Congress in opposition to the legislation. Near the end of the recording, these words can be heard:

> Write those letters now; call your friends and tell them to write them. If you don't, this program, I promise you, will pass just as surely as the sun will come up tomorrow. And behind it will come other federal programs that will invade every area of freedom as we have known it in this country. Until one day ... we will awake to find that we have socialism. And if you don't do this, and I don't do it, one of these days you and I are going to spend our sunset years telling our children and our children's children what it was like in America when men were free. (As quoted in Max Skidmore, *Medicare and the American Rhetoric of Reconciliation.* Tuscaloosa: University of Alabama Press, 1970, 138.)

The words are made all the more interesting by the fact that the voice on the recording, easily recognizable three decades after the recording was made, was that of Ronald Reagan.

In addition to establishing Titles XVIII and XIX, the Social Security Act Amendments of 1965 also amended Title V to authorize grant funds for maternal and child health and crippled children's services. These amendments also authorized grants for training professional personnel for the care of crippled children.

P.L. 89-239, the *Heart Disease, Cancer and Stroke Amendments,* amended the Public Health Act (see the 1944 P.L. 78-410) to establish a nationwide network of Regional Medical Programs. This legislation was intended to "assist in combating heart disease, cancer, stroke, and related diseases." Through its provisions, regional cooperative programs were established among medical schools, hospitals, and research institutions to foster research, training, continuing education, and demonstrations of patient care practices related to heart disease, cancer, and stroke.

P.L. 89-272, the *Clean Air Act Amendments of 1965*, amended the original Clean Air Act (see the 1963 P.L. 88-206) to provide for federal regulation of motor vehicle exhaust and to establish a program of federal research support and grants-in-aid in the area of solid waste disposal.

P.L. 89-290, the *Health Professions Educational Assistance Amendments*, amended the original act (see the 1963 P.L. 88-129) to provide further support "to improve the quality of schools of medicine, dentistry, osteopathy, optometry, and podiatry." The law expanded the availability of student loans and introduced a provision whereby 50 percent of a professional's student loan could be forgiven in exchange for practice in a designated shortage area.

1966

P.L. 89-794, the *Economic Opportunity Act Amendments*, amended the Economic Opportunity Act (see the 1964 P.L. 88-452) to establish Office of Economic Opportunity neighborhood health centers. Located especially in impoverished sections of cities and rural areas, these centers provided poor people a comprehensive range of ambulatory health services. By the early 1970s approximately 100 centers were to have been established under this program.

P.L. 89-564, the *Highway Safety Act*, sought to improve the nation's system of highways in order to make them safer for users.

P.L. 89-642, the *Child Nutrition Act*, established a federal program of support, including research, for child nutrition. A key component of the legislation was its authorization of the school breakfast program.

P.L. 89-749, the *Comprehensive Health Planning Act* (or the Partnership for Health Act), which amended the Public Health Service Act (see the 1944 P.L. 78-410), was intended "to promote and assist in the extension and improvement of comprehensive health planning and public health services, [and] to provide for a more effective use of available Federal funds for such planning and services . . . ." This legislation sought to promote comprehensive planning for health facilities, services, and personnel within the framework of a federal-state-local partnership. It also gave states greater flexibility in the use of their grants-in-aid for public health services through block grants.

The law, in Section 314a, authorized grants to states for the development of comprehensive state health planning; and, in Section 314b, authorized grants to public or nonprofit organizations "for developing comprehensive regional, metropolitan area or other local area plans for coordination of existing and planned health services." State planning agencies created or designated under this legislation became known as "A" agencies or as "314a" agencies. Within states, the other planning agencies created or designated under this legislation became known as "B" or "areawide" or "314b" agencies.

P.L. 89-751, the *Allied Health Professions Personnel Training Act*, provided grant support for the training of allied health professionals. The legislation was patterned after the 1963 Health Professions Education Assistance Act (see P.L. 88-129).

1967

P.L. 90-148, the *Air Quality Act*, amended the Clean Air Act (see the 1963 P.L. 88-206) "to authorize planning grants to air pollution control agencies; expand research provisions relating to fuels and vehicles; provide for interstate air pollution control agencies or commissions; authorize the establishment of air quality standards; and for other purposes." The act provided for each state to establish air quality standards depending on local conditions, but a minimum air quality was to be ensured through federal review of the states' standards.

P.L. 90-31, the *Mental Health Amendments*, amended the Mental Retardation Facilities and Community Mental Health Centers Construction Act (see the 1963 P.L. 88-164) to extend the program of construction grants for community mental health centers. The legislation also amended the term "construction" so that it covered acquisition of existing buildings.

P.L. 90-174, the *Clinical Laboratory Improvement Act*, amended the Public Health Service Act (see the 1944 P.L. 78-410) to provide for the regulation of laboratories in interstate commerce by the Centers for Disease Control through processes of licensure, standards setting, and proficiency testing.

P.L. 90-189, the *Flammable Fabrics Act*, was part of government's early efforts to rid the environment of hazards to human health. The legislation sought to regulate the manufacture and marketing of flammable fabrics.

P.L. 90-170, the *Mental Retardation Amendments*, amended the Mental Retardation Facilities and Community Mental Health Centers Construction Act (see the 1963 P.L. 88-164) to extend the program of construction grants for university-affiliated and community-based facilities for the mentally retarded. The legislation also authorized a new program of grants for the education of physical educators and recreation workers who would be prepared to work with mentally retarded and other handicapped children and for research in these areas.

P.L. 90-174, the *Partnership for Health Amendments*, amended the Partnership for Health Act (see the 1966 P.L. 89-749) by extending the program and by requiring that the interests of local governments be represented in areawide planning agencies.

P.L. 90-248, the *Social Security Amendments of 1967*, represented the first of many modifications to the Medicare and Medicaid programs established by the Social Security Amendments of 1965 (see the P.L. 89-97). Coming two years after their establishment, this legislation provided expanded coverage for such things as durable medical equipment for use in the home, podiatrist services for nonroutine foot care, outpatient physical therapy, and the addition of a lifetime reserve of 60 days of coverage for inpatient hospital care over and above the original coverage for up to 90 days during any spell of illness. In addition, certain payment rules were modified in favor of providers. For example, payment of full reasonable charges for radiologist's and pathologist's services provided to inpatients were authorized under one modification.

This law also sought to raise the quality of care provided in nursing homes by establishing a number of conditions that had to be met by nursing homes wanting to participate in the Medicare and Medicaid programs. There was also a provision for limiting the federal participation in medical assistance payments to families whose income did not exceed 133 percent of the income limit for Aid to Families With Dependent Children (AFDC) payments in any state.

1968

P.L. 90-490, the *Health Manpower Act*, extended previous programs of support for the training of health professionals (see the 1963 P.L. 88-129 and the 1964 P.L. 88-581), in effect authorizing formula institutional grants for training all health professionals.

1969

P.L. 91-173, the *Federal Coal Mine Health and Safety Act*, was intended to help secure and improve the health and safety of coal miners.

P.L. 91-190, the *National Environmental Policy Act of 1969*, was enacted "To declare a national policy which will encourage productive and enjoyable harmony between man and his environment; to promote efforts which will prevent or eliminate damage to the environment and biosphere and stimulate the health and welfare of man . . . . " This law established the Council on Environmental Quality, created to advise the president on environmental matters. The legislation required that environmental impact statements be prepared prior to the initiation of major federal actions.

1970

P.L. 91-224, the *Water Quality Improvement Act*, a very comprehensive water pollution law, included among its numerous provisions those relating to oil pollution by vessels and on- and offshore oil wells, hazardous polluting substances other than oil, pollution from sewage from vessels, and for training people to work in the operation and maintenance of water treatment facilities. Perhaps its most important provisions pertain to the procedures whereby all federal agencies must deal with water pollution, including requirements for cooperation among the various agencies.

P.L. 91-296, the *Medical Facilities Construction and Modernization Amendments*, amended the Hill-Burton Act (see the 1946 P.L. 79-725) by extending the program and by initiating a new program of project grants for emergency rooms, communications networks, and medical transportation systems.

P.L. 91-464, the *Communicable Disease Control Amendments*, amended the Public Health Service Act (see the 1944 P.L. 78-410), which had established the Communicable Disease Center (CDC), by renaming the CDC the Centers for Disease Control. The legislation also broadened the functions of the CDC beyond its traditional focus on communicable or infectious diseases (e.g., tuberculosis, venereal disease, rubella, measles, Rh disease, poliomyelitis, diphtheria, tetanus, and whooping cough) to include concern with other preventable conditions, including malnutrition.

P.L. 91-513, the *Comprehensive Drug Abuse Prevention and Control Act*, provided for special project grants for drug abuse and drug dependence treatment programs and grants for programs and activities related to drug education.

P.L. 91-572, the *Family Planning Services and Population Research Act*, established the Office of Population Affairs and added Title X, Population Research and Voluntary Family Planning Programs, to the Public Health Service Act (see the 1944 P.L. 78-410). The legislation authorized a range of project, formula, training, and research grants and contracts to support family planning programs and services, except for abortion.

P.L. 91-596, the *Occupational Safety and Health Act* (OSHA), established an extensive federal program of standard-setting and enforcement activities that were intended to ensure healthful and safe workplaces.

P.L. 91-601, the *Poison Prevention Packaging Act*, required that most drugs be dispensed in containers designed to be difficult for children to open.

P.L. 91-604, the *Clean Air Amendments of 1970*, was enacted because Congress became dissatisfied with progress toward control and abatement of air pollution under the Air Quality Act of 1967 (see the 1967 P.L. 90-148). This law took away the power of the states to establish different air quality standards in different air quality control regions. States were required by this legislation to achieve national air quality standards within each of their regions.

P.L. 91-616, the *Comprehensive Alcohol Abuse and Alcoholism Prevention, Treatment, and Rehabilitation Act*, established the National Institute of Alcohol Abuse and Alcoholism. The law provided a separate statutory base for programs and activities related to alcohol abuse and alcoholism. The legislation also provided a comprehensive program of aid to states and localities in their efforts addressed to combating alcohol abuse and alcoholism.

P.L. 91-623, the *Emergency Health Personnel Act*, amended the Public Health Service Act (see the 1944 P.L. 78-410) to permit the Secretary of DHEW (now DHHS) to assign commissioned officers and other health personnel of the U.S. Public Health Service to areas of the country experiencing critical shortages of health personnel. This legislation also established the National Health Service Corps.

P.L. 91-695, the *Lead-Based Paint Poisoning Prevention Act*, represented a specific attempt to address the problem of lead-based paint poisoning through a program of grants to the states to aid them in their efforts to combat this problem.

1971

P.L. 92-157, the *Comprehensive Health Manpower Training Act*, was, at the time of its enactment, the most comprehensive health personnel legislation yet enacted. The legislation replaced institutional formula grants with a new system of capitation grants through which health professions schools received fixed sums of money for each of their students (contingent on increasing first-year enrollments). Loan provisions were broadened so that 85 percent of education loans could be cancelled by health professionals who practiced in designated personnel shortage areas. The legislation also established the National Health Manpower Clearinghouse and the Secretary of DHEW (now DHHS) was directed to make every effort to provide to counties without physicians at least one National Health Service Corps physician.

1972

P.L. 92-294, the *National Sickle Cell Anemia Control Act*, authorized grants and contracts to support screening, treatment, counseling, information and education programs, and research related to sickle cell anemia.

P.L. 92-574, the *Noise Control Act*, much like the earlier Clean Air Act (see the 1963 P.L. 88-206) and the Flammable Fabrics Act (see the 1967 P.L. 90-189), continued government's efforts to rid the environment of harmful influences on human health.

P.L. 92-303, the *Federal Coal Mine Health and Safety Amendments*, amended the earlier Federal Coal Mine Health and Safety Act (see the 1969 P.L. 91-173) to provide financial benefits and other assistance to coalminers who were afflicted with black lung disease.

P.L. 92-426, the *Uniformed Services Health Professions Revitalization Act*, established the Uniformed Services University of the Health Sciences. The legislation provided for this educational institution to be operated under the auspices of the U.S. Department of Defense in Bethesda, Maryland. The legislation also created the Armed Forces Health Professions Scholarship Program.

P.L. 92-433, the *National School Lunch and Child Nutrition Amendments*, amended the Child Nutrition Act (see the 1966 P.L. 89-642) to add support for the provison of nutritious diets for pregnant and lactating women and for infants and children (the WIC program).

P.L. 92-573, the *Consumer Product Safety Act*, established the Consumer Product Safety Commission. The commission was created to develop safety standards and regulations for consumer products. Under provisons of the legislation, the administration of existing related legislation, including the Flammable Fabrics Act, the Hazardous Substances Act, and the Poison Prevention Packaging Act, was transferred to the commission.

P.L. 92-603, the *Social Security Amendments of 1972*, amended the Social Security Act (see the 1935 P.L. 74-271) to make several significant changes in the Medicare program. These amendments marked an important shift in the operation of the Medicare program as efforts were undertaken to help control its growing costs. Over the bitter opposition of organized medicine, the legislation established Professional Standards Review Organizations (PSROs) that were to monitor both the quality of services provided to Medicare beneficiaries as well as the medical necessity for the services.

One provision limited payments for capital expenditures by hospitals that had been disapproved by state or local planning agencies. Another provision authorized a program of grants and contracts to conduct experiments and demonstrations related to achieving increased economy and efficiency in the provision of health services. Some of the specifically targeted areas of these studies were to be prospective reimbursement, the requirement that patients spend three days in the hospital prior to admission to a skilled nursing home, the potential benefits of ambulatory surgery centers, payment for the services of physician's assistants and nurse practitioners, and the use of clinical psychologists.

Coincident with these and other cost-containment amendments, several cost-increasing changes were also made in the Medicare program by this legislation. Notably, persons who were eligible for cash benefits under the disability provisions of the Social Security Act for at least 24 months were made eligible for medical benefits under the program. In addition, persons who were insured under Social Security, as well as their dependents, who required hemodialysis or renal transplantation for chronic renal disease were defined as disabled for the purpose of having them covered under the Medicare program for the costs of treating their end-stage renal disease (ESRD). The inclusion of coverage for the disabled and ESRD patients in 1972 was an extraordinarily expensive change in the Medicare program. In addition, certain less costly but still expensive additional coverages were extended, including chiropractic services and speech pathology services.

P.L. 92-714, the *National Cooley's Anemia Control Act*, authorized grants and contracts to support screening, treatment, counseling, information and education programs, and research related to Cooley's Anemia.

1973

P.L. 93-154, the *Emergency Medical Services Systems Act*, provided aid to states and localities to assist them in developing coordinated Emergency Medical Service (EMS) Systems.

P.L. 93-222, the *Health Maintenance Organization Act*, amended the Public Health Service Act (see the 1944 P.L. 78-410) to "provide assistance and encouragement for the establishment and expansion of health maintenance organizations . . . . " The legislation, which added a new title, XIII, Health Maintenance Organizations, to the Public Health Service Act, authorized a program of grants, loans, and loan guarantees to support the conduct of feasibility and development studies and initial operations for new HMOs.

P.L. 93-29, the *Older Americans Act*, established the National Clearinghouse for Information on Aging and created the Federal Council on Aging. The legislation also authorized funds to establish gerontology centers and provided grants for training and research related to the field of aging.

1974

P.L. 93-247, the *Child Abuse Prevention and Treatment Act*, created the National Center on Child Abuse and Neglect. The legislation authorized grants for research and demonstrations related to child abuse and neglect.

P.L. 93-270, the *Sudden Infant Death Syndrome Act*, added Part C, Sudden Infant Death Syndrome, to Title XI of the Public Health Service Act (see the 1944 P.L. 78-410). The legislation provided for the development of informational programs related to this syndrome for both public and professional audiences.

P.L. 93-406, the *Employee Retirement Income Security Act*, also known as ERISA, provided for the regulation of almost all pension and benefit plans for employees, including pensions, medical or hospital benefits, disability, and death benefits. The legislation provides for the regulation of many features of these benefit plans.

P.L. 93-296, *Research in Aging Act*, established the National Institute on Aging within the National Institutes of Health (NIH).

P.L. 93-344, the *Congressional Budget and Impoundment Act*, established the U.S. Congressional Budget Office (CBO). The nonpartison CBO conducts studies and analyses of the fiscal and budget implications of various decisions facing the Congress, including those related to health.

P.L. 93-360, the *Nonprofit Hospital Amendments*, amended the 1947 Labor-Management Relations Act (or the Taft-Hartley Act), to end the exclusion of nongovernmental nonprofit hospitals from the provisions of this act as well as from the earlier National Labor Relations Act of 1935 (or the Wagner Act). Both of these acts pertain to fair labor practices and collective bargaining.

P.L. 93-523, the *Safe Drinking Water Act*, required the Environmental Protection Agency (EPA) to establish national drinking water standards and to aid states and localities in the enforcement of these standards.

P.L. 93-641, the *National Health Planning and Resources Development Act*, amended the Public Health Service Act (see the 1944 P.L. 78-410) in an attempt "to assure the development of a national health policy and of effective state and area health planning and resource development programs, and for other purposes." The legislation added two new titles, XV and XVI, to the Public Health Service Act. These titles superseded and significantly modified the programs established under Sections 314a and 314b of Title III of the 1966 P.L. 89-749, the Comprehensive Health Planning Act (or the Partnership for Health Act), as well as the programs established under the Hill-Burton Act (see the 1946 P.L. 79-725).

The legislation essentially folded existing health planning activities into a new framework created by the legislation. The Secretary of DHEW (now DHHS) was to enter into an agreement with each state's governor for the designation of a State Health Planning and Development Agency (SHPDA). The states were to also establish State Health Coordinating Councils (SHCCs) to serve as advisors in setting overall state policy.

A network of local Health Systems Agencies (HSAs) covering the entire nation was established by the legislation. The HSAs were to: (1) improve the health of area residents; (2) increase the accessibility, acceptability, continuity, and quality of health services; and (3) restrain health care cost increases and prevent duplication of health care services and facilities. An important feature of the planning framework created by P.L. 93-641 was a provision that permitted the HSAs in states that had established certificate-of-need (CON) programs to conduct CON reviews and to make recommendations developed at the local level to the SHPDA.

Congress repealed this law in 1986 (effective 1 January 1987), leaving responsibility for the certificate-of-need programs entirely in the hands of the states.

P.L. 93-647, the *Social Security Amendments of 1974* (or the Social Services Amendments), amended the Social Security Act (see the 1935 P.L. 74-271) to consolidate existing federal-state social service programs into a block grant program that would permit a ceiling on federal matching funds while providing more flexibility to the states in providing certain social services. The legislation added a new title, XX, Grants to the States for Services, to the Social Security Act.

The goals of the legislation pertained to the prevention and remedy of neglect, abuse, or exploitation of children or adults, the preservation of families, and the avoidance of inappropriate institutional care by substituting community-based programs and services. Social services covered under this law included child care service; protective, foster, and day care services for children and adults; counseling; family planning services; homemaker services; and home-delivered meals.

1976

P.L. 94-295, the *Medical Devices Amendments*, amended the Federal Food, Drug and Cosmetic Act (see the 1938 P.L. 75-717) to strengthen the regulation of medical devices. This legislation was passed, after previous attempts had failed, amidst growing public concern with the adverse effects of such medical devices as the Dalcon Shield intrauterine device.

P.L. 94-317, *National Consumer Health Information and Health Promotion Act*, amended the Public Health Service Act (see the 1944 P.L. 78-410) to add Title XVII, Health Information and Promotion. The legislation authorized grants and contracts for research and community programs related to health information, health promotion, preventive health services, and education of the public in the appropriate use of health care services.

P.L. 94-437, the *Indian Health Care Improvement Act*, an extensive piece of legislation, was intended to fill existing gaps in the delivery of health care services to Native Americans.

P.L. 94-460, the *Health Maintenance Organization Amendments*, amended the Health Maintenance Organization Act (see the 1973 P.L. 93-222) to ease somewhat the requirements that had to be met for an HMO to become federally qualified. One provision, however, required that HMOs must be federally qualified if they were to receive reimbursement from the Medicare or Medicaid programs.

P.L. 94-469, the *Toxic Substances Control Act* (TSCA) sought to regulate chemical substances used in various production processes. The legislation defined chemical substances very broadly. The purpose of TSCA was to identify potentially harmful chemical substances before they were produced and entered the marketplace and, subsequently, the environment.

P.L. 94-484, the *Health Professions Educational Assistance Act*, extended the program of capitation grants to professional schools that had been established under the Comprehensive Health Manpower Training Act (see the 1971 P.L. 92-157). However, this legislation dropped the requirement that schools increase their first-year enrollments as a condition for receiving grants. Under this legislation, medical schools were required to have 50 percent of their graduates to enter residency programs in primary care by 1980. They were also required to reserve positions in their third-year classes for U.S. citizens who were studying medicine in foreign medical schools. However, under intense protest from medical schools, this provision was repealed in 1975.

1977

P.L. 95-142, the *Medicare-Medicaid Antifraud and Abuse Amendments*, amended the legislation governing the Medicare and Medicaid programs (see the 1965 P.L. 89-97) in an attempt to reduce fraud and abuse in the programs as a means to help contain their costs. Specific changes included strengthening criminal and civil penalties for fraud and abuse affecting the programs, modification in the operations of the PSROs, and the promulgation of uniform reporting systems and formats for hospitals and certain other health care organizations participating in the Medicare and Medicaid programs.

P.L. 95-210, the *Rural Health Clinic Services Amendments*, amended the legislation governing the Medicare and Medicaid programs (see the 1965 P.L. 89-97) to modify the categories of practitioners who could provide reimbursable services to Medicare and Medicaid beneficiaries, at least in rural settings. Under the provisions of this act, rural health clinics that did not routinely have physicians available on site could, if they met certain requirements regarding physician supervision of the clinic and review of services, be reimbursed for services provided by nurse practitioners and physician's assistants through the Medicare and Medicaid programs. This act also authorized certain demonstration projects in underserved urban areas for reimbursement of these nonphysician practitioners.

1978

P.L. 95-292, the *Medicare End-Stage Renal Disease Amendments*, further amended the legislation governing the Medicare program (see the 1965 P.L. 89-97) in an attempt to help control the program's costs. Since the addition of coverage for ESRD under the Social Security Amendments of 1972 (P.L. 92-603), the costs to the Medicare program had risen steadily and quickly. This legislation added incentives to encourage the use of home dialysis and the use of renal transplantation in ESRD.

The legislation also permitted the use of a variety of reimbursement methods for renal dialysis facilities. And it authorized funding for the conduct of studies of end-stage renal disease itself, especially studies incorporating possible cost reductions in treatment for this disease. It also directed the Secretary of DHEW (now DHHS) to establish areawide network coordinating councils to help plan for and review ESRD programs.

P.L. 95-559, the *Health Maintenance Organization Amendments,* further amended the Health Maintenance Organization Act (see the 1973 P.L. 93-222) to add a new program of loans and loan guarantees to support the acquisition of ambulatory care facilities and related equipment. The legislation also provided for support for a program of training for HMO administrators and medical directors and for providing technical assistance to HMOs in their developmental efforts.

1979

P.L. 96-79, the *Health Planning and Resources Development Amendments,* amended the National Health Planning and Resources Development Act (see the 1974 P.L. 93-641) to add provisions intended to foster competition within the health sector, to address the need to integrate mental health and alcoholism and drug abuse resources into health system plans, and to make several revisions in the certificate-of-need (CON) requirements.

1980

P.L. 96-398, the *Mental Health Systems Act,* extensively amended the Community Mental Health Centers program (see the 1970 P.L. 91-211) including provisions for the development and support of comprehensive state mental health systems. However, this legislation was almost completely superseded by the block grants to the states for mental health and alcohol and drug abuse that were provided under the Omnimbus Budget Reconciliation Act of 1981 (see P.L. 97-35).

P.L. 96-499, the *Omnibus Budget Reconciliation Act* (OBRA '80), contained in Title IX of the act the Medicare and Medicaid Amendments of 1980. These amendments made extensive modifications in the Medicare and Medicaid programs, with 57 separate sections pertaining to one or both of the programs. Many of the changes reflected continuing concern with the growing costs of the programs and were intended to help control these costs.

Examples of the changes that were specific to Medicare included removal of the 100 visits/year limitation on home health services and the requirement that patients pay a deductible for home care visits under Part B of the program. These changes were intended to encourage home care over more expensive institutional care. Another provision permitted small rural hospitals to use their beds as "swing beds" (alternating their use as acute or long-term care beds as needed) and authorized swing-bed demonstration projects for large and urban hospitals. An important change in the Medicaid program required the programs to pay for the services that the states had authorized nurse-midwives to perform.

P.L. 96-510, the *Comprehensive Environmental Response, Compensation and Liability Act* (CERCLA), established the Superfund program that intended to provide resources for the clean up of inactive hazardous waste dumps. The legislation assigned retroactive liability for the costs of cleaning up the dumps to their owners and operators as well as to the waste generators and transporters who had used the dump sites.

1981

P.L. 97-35, the *Omnibus Budget Reconciliation Act* (OBRA '81), in its Title XXI, Subtitles A, B, and C, contained further amendments to the Medicare and Medicaid programs. Just as in 1980, this legislation included extensive changes in the programs, with 46 sections pertaining to them. Enacted in the context of extensive efforts to reduce the federal budget, many of the provisions hit Medicare and Medicaid especially hard. For example, one provision eliminated the coverage of alcohol detoxification facility services, another removed the use of occupational therapy as a basis for initial entitlement to home health service, and yet another increased the Part B deductible.

In other provisions, OBRA '81 combined 20 existing categorical public health programs into four block grants. The block grants were: (1) Preventive Health and Health Services, which combined such previously categorical programs as rodent control, fluoridation, hypertension control, and rape crisis centers among others into one block grant to be distributed among the states by a formula based on population and other factors; (2) Alcohol Abuse, Drug Abuse, and Mental Health Block Grant, which combined existing programs created under the Community Mental Health Centers Act, the Mental Health Systems Act, the Comprehensive Alcohol Abuse and Alcoholism Prevention, Treatment, and Rehabilitation Act, and the Drug Abuse, Prevention, Treatment, and Rehabilitation Act; (3) Primary Care Block Grant, which consisted of the Community Health Centers; and (4) Maternal and Child Health Block Grant, which consolidated seven previously categorical grant programs from Title V of the Social Security Act and from the Public Health Services Act, including the maternal and child health and crippled children's programs, genetic disease service, adolescent pregnancy services, sudden infant death syndrome, hemophilia treatment, Supplemental Security Income (SSI) payments to disabled children, and lead-based poisoning prevention.

1982

P.L. 97-248, the *Tax Equity and Fiscal Responsibility Act* (TEFRA), made a number of important changes in the Medicare program. One provision added coverage for hospice services provided to Medicare beneficiaries. These benefits were extended later and are now an integral part of the Medicare program. However, the most important provisions, in terms of impact on the Medicare program, were those that sought to control the program's costs by setting limits on how much Medicare would reimburse hospitals on a per case basis and by limiting the annual rate of increase for Medicare's reasonable costs per discharge. These changes in reimbursement methodology represented fundamental changes in the Medicare program and reflected a dramatic shift in the nation's Medicare policy.

Another provision of TEFRA replaced PSROs, which had been established by the Social Security Amendments of 1972 (see the 1975 P.L. 92-603), with a new utilization and quality control program called peer review organizations (PROs). The TEFRA changes regarding the operation of the Medicare program were extensive, but they were only the harbinger of the most sweeping legislative changes in the history of the Medicare program the following year.

P.L. 97-414, the *Orphan Drug Act* (ODA), provided financial incentives for the development and marketing of orphan drugs, defined by the legislation to be drugs for the treatment of diseases or conditions affecting so few people that revenues from sales of the drugs would not cover their development costs.

1983

P.L. 98-21, the *Social Security Amendments of 1983*, another landmark in the evolution of the Medicare program, amended the legislation governing the program (see the 1965 P.L. 89-97) to initiate the Medicare prospective payment system (PPS). The legislation included provisions to base payment for hospital inpatient services on predetermined rates per discharge for diagnosis-related groups (DRGs). PPS was a major departure from the cost-based system of reimbursement that had been used in the Medicare program since its inception in 1965. The legislation also directed the administration to study physician payment reform options, a feature that was to later have significant impact (see the 1989 P.L. 101-239).

1984

P.L. 98-369, the *Deficit Reduction Act* (DEFRA), among many provisions, temporarily froze increases in physicians' fees paid under the Medicare program. Another provision in the legislation placed a specific limitation on the rate of increase in the DRG payment rates that the Secretary of DHHS could permit in the two subsequent years.

The legislation also established the Medicare Participating Physician and Supplier (PAR) program and created two classes of physicians in regard to their relationships to the Medicare program and outlined different reimbursement approaches for them depending on whether they were classified as "participating" or "nonparticipating." As part of this legislation, Congress mandated that the Office of Technology Assessment study alternative methods of paying for physician services so that the information could guide the reform of the Medicare program.

P.L. 98-417, the *Drug Price Competition and Patent Term Restoration Act*, provided brand name pharmaceutical manufacturers with patent term extensions. These extensions significantly increased manufacturers' opportunities for earning profits during the longer effective patent life (EPL) of their affected products.

P.L. 98-457, the *Child Abuse Amendments*, amended the Child Abuse Prevention and Treatment Act (see the 1974 P.L. 93-247) to involve Infant Care Review Committees in the medical decisions regarding the treatment of handicapped newborns, at least in hospitals with tertiary-level neonatal care units.

The legislation established treatment and reporting guidelines for severely disabled newborns, making it illegal to withold "medically indicated treatment" from newborns except when "in the treating physician's reasonable medical judgment, i) the infant is chronically and irreversibly comatose; ii) the provision of such treatment would merely prolong dying, not be effective in ameliorating or correcting all of the infant's life-threatening conditions, or otherwise be futile in terms of survival of the infant; or iii) the provision of such treatment would be virtually futile in terms of the survival of the infant and the treatment itself under such circumstances would be inhumane."

P.L. 98-507, the *National Organ Transplant Act*, made it illegal "to knowingly acquire, receive or otherwise transfer any human organ for valuable consideration for use in human transplantation if the transfer affects interstate commerce."

1985

P.L. 99-177, the *Emergency Deficit Reduction and Balanced Budget Act* (or the Gramm-Rudman-Hollins Act), established mandatory deficit reduction targets for the five subsequent fiscal years. Under provisions of the legislation, the required budget cuts would come equally from defense spending and from domestic programs that were not exempted. The Gramm-Rudman-Hollins Act had signficant impact on the Medicare program throughout the last half of the 1980s, as well as on other health programs such as community and migrant health centers, veteran and Native American health, health professions education, and the

National Institutes of Health. Among other things, this legislation led to substantial cuts in Medicare payments to hospitals and physicians.

P.L. 99-272, the *Consolidated Omnibus Budget Reconciliation Act* (COBRA '85), contained a number of provisions that impacted on the Medicare program. Hospitals that served a disproportionate share of poor patients received an adjustment in their PPS payments; hospice care was made a permanent part of the Medicare program and states were given the ability to provide hospice services under the Medicaid program; fiscal year 1986 PPS payment rates were frozen at 1985 levels through 1 May 1986 and increased 0.5 of a percent for the remainder of the year; payment to hospitals for the indirect costs of medical education were modified; and a schedule to phase out payment of a return on equity to proprietary hospitals was established.

This legislation established the Physician Payment Review Commission (PPRC) to advise Congress on physician payment policies for the Medicare program. The legislation also required that the PPRC advise Congress and the Secretary of the DHHS regarding the development of a resource-based relative value scale for physician services.

Under another of COBRA's important provisions, employers were required to continue health insurance for employees and their dependents who would otherwise lose their eligibility for the coverage due to reduced hours of work or termination of their employment.

1986

P.L. 99-509, the *Omnibus Budget Reconciliation Act* (OBRA '86), altered the PPS payment rate for hospitals once again and reduced payment amounts for capital-related costs by 3.5 percent for part of fiscal year 1987, by 7 percent for fiscal year 1988, and by 10 percent for fiscal year 1989. In addition, certain adjustments were made in the manner in which "outlier" or atypical cases were reimbursed.

The legislation established further limits to balance billing by physicians providing services to Medicare clients by setting "maximum allowable actual charges" (MAACs) for physicians who did not particiapte in the PAR program (see the Deficit Reduction Act of 1984, P.L. 98-369). In another provision intended to realize savings for the Medicare program, OBRA '86 directed the DHHS to use the concept of "inherent reasonableness" to reduce payments for cataract surgery as well as for anesthesia during the surgery.

P.L. 99-660, the *Omnibus Health Act*, contained provisions to significantly liberalize coverage under the Medicaid program. Using family income up to the federal poverty line as a criterion, this change permitted states to offer coverage to all pregnant women, infants up to one year of age, and by using a phase-in schedule, children up to five years of age.

One part of this omnibus health legislation was the National Childhood Vaccine Injury Act. This law established a federal vaccine injury compensation system. Under provisions of the legislation, parties injured by vaccines would be limited to awards of income losses plus $250,000 for pain and suffering or death.

Another important part of the omnibus health legislation of 1986 was the Health Care Quality Improvement Act. This law provided immunity from private damage lawsuits under federal or state law for "any professional review action" so long as that action followed standards set out in the legislation. This afforded members of peer review committees protection from most damage suits that might have been filed by physicians whom they disciplined. The law also mandated creation of a national data bank through which information on physician licensure actions, sanctions by boards of medical examiners, malpractice claims paid, and professional review actions that adversely affect the clinical privileges of physicians could be provided to authorized persons and organizations.

1987

P.L. 100-177, the *National Health Service Corps Amendments*, reauthorized the National Health Service Corps (NHSC), which had been created under a provision of the Emergency Health Personnel Act of 1970 (see P.L. 91-623).

P.L. 100-203, the *Omnibus Budget Reconciliation Act* (OBRA '87), contained a number of provisions that directly impacted on the Medicare program. It required the Secretary of the DHHS to update the wage index used in calculating hospital PPS payments by 1 October 1990 and to do so at least every three years thereafter. It also required the Secretary to study and report to Congress on the criteria being used by the Medicare program to identify referral hospitals. Deepening the reductions established by OBRA '86, one provision of the act reduced payment amounts for capital-related costs by 12 percent for fiscal year 1988 and by 15 percent for 1989.

Regarding payments to physicians for services provided to Medicare clients, the legislation reduced fees for 12 sets of "overvalued" procedures. It also allowed higher fee increases for primary care than for other physician services and increased the fee differential between participating and nonparticipating physicians (see the 1984 P.L. 98-369).

The legislation also contained a number of provisions that impacted on the Medicaid program. Key among these, the law provided additional options for children and pregnant women, and required states to cover eligible children up to age six with an option for allowing coverage up to age eight. The distinction between skilled nursing facilities (SNFs) and intermediate care facilities (ICFs) was eliminated. The legislation contained a number of provisions intended to enhance the quality of services provided in nursing homes, including requirements that nursing homes enhance the quality of life of each resident and operate quality assurance programs.

1988

P.L. 100-360, the *Medicare Catastrophic Coverage Act*, provided the largest expansion of the benefits covered under the Medicare program since its establishment in 1965 (see P.L. 89-97). Among other things, provisions of this legislation added coverage for outpatient prescription drugs and respite care and placed a cap on out-of-pocket spending for copayment costs for covered services by the elderly.

The legislation included provisions that would have the new benefits phased in over a four-year period and paid for by premiums charged to Medicare program enrollees. Thirty-seven percent of the costs were to be covered by a fixed monthly premium paid by all enrollees and the remainder of the costs were to be covered by an income-related supplemental premium that was, in effect, an income tax surtax that would apply to fewer than half of the enrollees. Under intense pressure from many of their elderly constituents and their interest groups who objected to having to pay additional premiums or the income tax surtax, Congress repealed P.L. 100-360 in 1989 without implementing most of its provisions.

P.L. 100-578, the *Clinical Laboratory Improvement Amendments*, amended the Clinical Laboratory Improvement Act (see the 1967 P.L. 90-174) to extend and modify government's ability to regulate clinical laboratories.

P.L. 100-607, the *National Organ Transplant Amendments*, amended the National Organ Transplant Act (see the 1986 P.L. 98-507) to extend the prohibition against the sale of human organs to the organs and other body parts of human fetuses.

P.L. 100-647, the *Technical and Miscellaneous Revenue Act*, directed the Physician Payment Review Commission (see the 1985 P.L. 99-272) to consider policies for moderating the rate of increase in expenditures for physician services in the Medicare program and for reducing the utilization of these services.

P.L. 100-582, the *Medical Waste Tracking Act*, was enacted in response to the highly publicized incidents of used and discarded syringes and needles washing up on the shores of a number of states in the eastern United States in the summer of 1988. The legislation itself was rather limited in that it focused on the tracking of medical wastes from their origin to their disposal rather than broader regulation of transportation and disposal of these wastes.

1989

P.L. 101-239, the *Omnibus Budget Reconciliation Act* (OBRA '89), included provisions for minor, primarily technical, changes in the PPS and a provision to extend coverage for mental health benefits and add coverage for Pap smears. Small adjustments were made in the disproportionate share regulations, and the 15 percent capital-related payment reduction established in OBRA '87 was continued in OBRA '89. Another provision required the Secretary of DHHS to update the wage index annually in a budget-neutral manner beginning in fiscal year 1993.

As part of the OBRA '89 legislation, the Health Care Financing Administration (HCFA) was directed to begin implementing a resource-based relative value scale (RBRVS) for reimbursing physicians under the Medicare program on 1 January 1992. The new system was to be phased in over a four-year period beginning in 1992.

Another important provision in this legislation initiated the establishment of the Agency for Health Care Policy and Research (AHCPR). This agency succeeded the National Center for Health Services Research and Technology Assessment (NCHSR). The new agency was created to conduct and to foster the conduct of studies of health care quality, effectiveness, and efficiency. In particular, the agency was to conduct and to foster the conduct of studies on the outcomes of medical treatments and provide technical assistance to groups seeking to develop practice guidelines.

1990

P.L. 101-508, the *Omnibus Budget Reconciliation Act* (OBRA '90), contained the Patient Self-Determination Act, which required health care institutions participating in the Medicare and Medicaid programs to provide all their patients with written information on policies regarding self-determination and living wills. The institutions were also required under this legislation to inquire whether patients had advance medical directives and to document the replies in the patients' medical records.

The legislation made additional minor changes in the PPS, including further adjustments in the wage index calculation and in the disproportionate share regulations. Regarding the wage index, one provision required ProPAC (the Prospective Payment Assessment Commission), which was established by the 1983 Social Security Amendments (see P.L. 98-21), to help guide the Congress and the Secretary of DHHS on implementing the PPS to further study the available data on wages by occupational category and to develop recommendations on modifying the wage index to account for occupational mix.

The legislation also included a provision that continued the 15 percent capital-related payment reduction that was established in OBRA '87 and continued in OBRA '89 and another provision that made the reduced teaching adjustment payment established in OBRA '87 permanent. One of its more important provisions provided a five-year deficit reduction plan that was to reduce total Medicare outlays by more than $43 billion between fiscal years 1991 and 1995.

P.L. 101-336, the *Americans With Disabilities Act* (or ADA), provided a broad range of protections for the disabled, in effect combining protections contained in the Civil Rights Act of 1964, the Rehabilitation Act of 1973, and the Civil Rights Restoration Act of 1988. The central goal of the legislation was independence for the disabled, in effect to assist them in being self-supporting and able to lead independent lives.

P.L. 101-629, the *Safe Medical Devices Act*, further amended the Federal Food, Drug and Cosmetic Act (see the 1938 P.L. 75-717) and the subsequent Medical Devices Amendments of 1976 (see the P.L. 94-295) to require institutions that use medical devices to report device-related problems to the manufacturers and/or to the FDA. Reportable problems include any incident in which any medical device may have caused or contributed to any person's death, serious illness, or serious injury.

P.L. 101-649, the *Immigration and Nationality Act of 1990*, restructured with minor modifications the medical exclusion scheme for screening people who desired to immigrate to the United States that had been in use since the enactment of the Immigration and Nationality Act of 1952 (see P.L. 82-414).

1993

P.L. 103-43, the *National Institutes of Health Revitalization Act*, contained provisions for a number of structural and budgetary changes in the operation of the NIH. It also set forth guidelines for the conduct of research on transplantation of human fetal tissue and added HIV infection to the list of excludable conditions covered by the Immigration and Nationality Act (see the 1990 P.L. 101-649).

P.L. 103-66, the *Omnibus Budget Reconciliation Act* (OBRA '93), established an all-time record, five-year cut in Medicare funding and included a number of other changes affecting the Medicare program. For example, the legislation included provisions to end return on equity (ROE) payments for capital to proprietary SNFs and reduced the previously established rate of increase in payment rates for care provided in hospices. In addition, the legislation cut laboratory fees drastically by changing the reimbursement formula and froze payments for durable medical equipment, parenteral and enteral services, and for orthotics and prosthetics in fiscal years 1994 and 1995.

OBRA '93 contained the Comprehensive Childhood Immunization Act, which provided $585 million to support the provision of vaccines for children eligible for Medicaid, children who do not have health insurance, and for Native American children.

Index

About the Author

Beaufort B. Longest, Jr., Ph.D., is Professor of Health Services Administration in the Graduate School of Public Health, Professor of Business Administration in the Katz Graduate School of Business, and the founding Director of the Health Policy Institute at the University of Pittsburgh. Previously, he was on the faculties of Georgia State University and of the Kellogg Graduate School of Management at Northwestern University. A Fellow of the American College of Healthcare Executives, his research on issues of health management and policy has stimulated substantial external funding support and has resulted in numerous publications. He is co-author of *Managing Health Services Organizations*, Third Edition, one of the most widely used textbooks in graduate health management programs, and is currently revising for the fifth time his *Management Practices for the Health Professional*. He consults widely with associations, government agencies, health care organizations, and universities on health policy and management issues.